Department of Veterans Affairs
Health Services Research & Development Service

Evidence-based Synthesis Program

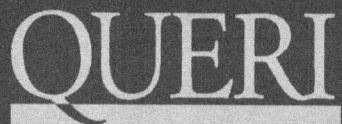

Suicide Prevention Interventions and Referral/Follow-up Services: A Systematic Review

March 2012

Prepared for:
Department of Veterans Affairs
Veterans Health Administration
Quality Enhancement Research Initiative
Health Services Research & Development Service
Washington, DC 20420

Prepared by:
Evidence-based Synthesis Program (ESP) Center
Portland VA Medical Center
Portland, OR
Devan Kansagara, M.D., M.C.R., Director

Investigators:
Principal Investigator:
Maya Elin O'Neil, Ph.D., M.S.

Co-Investigators and Research Associates:
Kimberly Peterson, M.S.
Allison Low, B.A.
Susan Carson, M.P.H.
Lauren M Denneson, Ph.D.
Elizabeth Haney, M.D.
Paulo Shiroma, M.D.
Devan Kansagara, M.D., M.C.R.

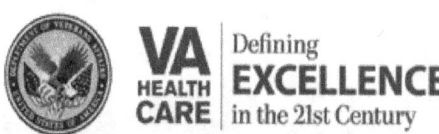

PREFACE

Quality Enhancement Research Initiative's (QUERI) Evidence-based Synthesis Program (ESP) was established to provide timely and accurate syntheses of targeted healthcare topics of particular importance to Veterans Affairs (VA) managers and policymakers, as they work to improve the health and healthcare of Veterans. The ESP disseminates these reports throughout VA.

QUERI provides funding for four ESP Centers and each Center has an active VA affiliation. The ESP Centers generate evidence syntheses on important clinical practice topics, and these reports help:

- develop clinical policies informed by evidence,
- guide the implementation of effective services to improve patient outcomes and to support VA clinical practice guidelines and performance measures, and
- set the direction for future research to address gaps in clinical knowledge.

In 2009, the ESP Coordinating Center was created to expand the capacity of QUERI Central Office and the four ESP sites by developing and maintaining program processes. In addition, the Center established a Steering Committee comprised of QUERI field-based investigators, VA Patient Care Services, Office of Quality and Performance, and Veterans Integrated Service Networks (VISN) Clinical Management Officers. The Steering Committee provides program oversight, guides strategic planning, coordinates dissemination activities, and develops collaborations with VA leadership to identify new ESP topics of importance to Veterans and the VA healthcare system.

Comments on this evidence report are welcome and can be sent to Nicole Floyd, ESP Coordinating Center Program Manager, at nicole.floyd@va.gov.

Recommended citation: O'Neil ME, Peterson K, Low A, Carson S, Denneson LM, Haney E, Shiroma P and Kansagara D. Suicide Prevention Interventions and Referral/Follow-up Services: A Systematic Review. VA-ESP Project #05-225; 2012.

TABLE OF CONTENTS

EXECUTIVE SUMMARY

INTRODUCTION

Suicide is the tenth leading cause of death in the United States (US), with nearly 100 suicides occurring each day and over 36,000 dying by suicide each year.[1] Among Veterans and current military, suicide is a national public health concern. Recent estimates suggest current or former military represent 20 percent of all known suicides in the US[2] and the rate of suicides among Veterans utilizing Veterans Health Administration (VHA) services is estimated to be higher than the general population.[3] The enormity of the problem has led to several major public health initiatives and a growth in research funding for suicide prevention.[4-7]

Despite recent suicide prevention efforts, the suicide rate in the US has changed relatively little over the past 100 years.[8] The body of research on suicide prevention approaches has been reviewed previously by Gaynes and colleagues,[9] and Mann and colleagues,[9, 10] and recent, similar work exists in the form of draft self-harm guidelines from the National Institute for Health and Clinical Excellence (NICE) in 2011.[11] As requested by the Veterans Affairs (VA)/Department of Defense (DoD) Evidence Based Practice Working Group (EBPWG) on suicide prevention, we examined recent research on suicidal self-directed violence as defined by Crosby et al. 2011.[12] We update the work of Gaynes et al. and Mann et al. by systematically reviewing relevant literature that was not included in either report, and was published in 2005 through November 18, 2011. Though the focus of the report is on suicide prevention, we include as outcomes any type of suicidal self-directed violence, defined as "Behavior that is self-directed and deliberately results in injury or the potential for injury to oneself. There is evidence, whether implicit or explicit, of suicidal intent."[12, 13]

The key questions were:

Key Question #1. What is the effectiveness of specific interventions for reducing rates of suicidal self-directed violence in military and/or Veteran populations?

Key Question #2. What lessons can be learned from suicidal self-directed violence prevention intervention research conducted outside of Veteran or military settings that can be applied to Veteran and/or military populations?

Key Question #3. What is the effectiveness of referral and follow-up services (e.g., strategies designed to provide referrals, improve referral follow-through and attendance, etc.) for reducing rates of suicidal self-directed violence in military and/or Veteran populations?

Key Question #4. What lessons can be learned from research on suicidal self-directed violence referral and follow-up services conducted outside of Veteran or military settings that can be applied to Veteran and/or military populations?

METHODS

The VA/DoD suicide prevention Evidence Based Practice Workgroup (EBPWG) requested a systematic review of literature related to suicidal self-directed violence published since two prior reports on the topic by Mann et al. and Gaynes et al.[9, 10] The workgroup requested a review focused on countries and populations of interest due to their similarity to US Veteran and military populations. Though a previous systematic review was conducted by Shekelle and colleagues in 2009,[14] the EBPWG requested that the current review include studies of pharmacotherapy and psychotherapy interventions, which were largely excluded from this previous report; and, therefore, we used the end search date from the Mann et al. review as the starting point for the current search. We identified relevant systematic reviews and controlled trials by searching PubMed, PsycINFO, the Cochrane Database of Systematic Reviews®, and the Cochrane Central Register of Controlled Trials® from 2005 to November 18, 2011. We used suicide and related terminology, and included interventions, military, Veterans as search terms (Appendix A). We limited the search to peer-reviewed articles involving human subjects and published in the English language that were not included in the previously published systematic reviews on the topic.[9, 10] We also report results from these two older systematic reviews, as well as results from a draft systematic review on self-harm,[11] comparing and combining findings across the three reports to the findings in this current report. Additional citations were identified from reference lists, consultation with content experts, and web sources. Titles, abstracts, and articles were reviewed by doctoral level investigators and project research associates trained in the critical analysis of literature; all articles were reviewed in duplicate. Quality assessment of all included primary studies and systematic reviews was performed in duplicate by investigators and research associates. We assessed study quality of systematic reviews using Oxman and Guyatt criteria.[15] We assessed the risk of bias of primary studies using the tool described in version 5.1.0 of the *Cochrane Handbook for Systematic Reviews of Interventions*.[16] Data on study characteristics, patient characteristics, and outcomes were extracted by trained research associates under the supervision of the Principal Investigator, a VA clinical psychologist. All data were narratively summarized.

DATA SYNTHESIS

We constructed evidence tables showing study, patient, and intervention characteristics; methodological quality; and outcomes, organized by key question, intervention type, and comparison group. We analyzed studies to compare their characteristics, methods, and findings. We graded strength of evidence based on the guidance established for the Evidence-based Practice Center (EPC) Program of the Agency for Healthcare Research and Quality (AHRQ).[17] We compiled a summary of findings for each question based on qualitative and semi-quantitative synthesis of the findings. We identified and highlighted findings from VA and DoD populations.

PEER REVIEW

A draft version of this report was reviewed by eight technical experts, as well as clinical leadership. Reviewer comments were addressed and our responses were incorporated in the final report (Appendix AA).

RESULTS

We reviewed 16,518 titles and abstracts from the electronic and hand searches. Applying our inclusion/exclusion criteria eliminated studies published prior to 2005; studies that did not report suicidal self-directed violence as an outcome; studies that were not randomized controlled trials

(RCTs); and studies conducted in countries other than Australia, Canada, New Zealand, the United Kingdom, and the United States. We rejected 16,110 at the abstract level, and performed a more detailed full-text review on 408 articles. From these, we identified 38 RCTs (reported in 47 publications) and 23 systematic reviews (reported in 25 publications) that addressed at least one of the key questions.

We classified studies as pharmacotherapy interventions, psychotherapy interventions, or referral and follow-up services. We defined interventions as interventions designed to treat a condition, symptom, or behavior. Referral and follow-up services were any services that were provided to patients that were primarily designed to facilitate access to interventions rather than treat a condition, symptom, or behavior. Because many interventions include components designed to increase adherence and attendance, we classified any study describing an intervention component as an "intervention" study rather than a "referral and follow-up services" study even if it also included components of referral and follow-up services. Therefore, the studies designated as referral and follow-up services were described by the authors as solely designed to increase access to, attendance at, and adherence to other interventions not included in the study design.

Key Question #1. What is the effectiveness of specific interventions for reducing rates of suicidal self-directed violence in military and/or Veteran populations?

We found no RCTs of self-directed violence prevention interventions in military and/or VA health care settings.

Key Question #2. What lessons can be learned from suicidal self-directed violence prevention intervention research conducted outside of Veteran or military settings that can be applied to Veteran and/or military populations?

Pharmacotherapy Results

Findings from other systematic reviews with similar key questions report that pharmacotherapy findings are based on few studies with limited sample sizes, some methodological quality concerns, and short term follow-up assessment periods;[9-11] therefore, pharmacotherapy findings should be interpreted with caution. All three reports found that available evidence from antidepressant trials does not show a benefit for reducing suicide, but caution that rates of suicide may have been too low to detect differences. Although observational studies show a correlation between increasing prescription rates and decreasing suicide rates, this evidence is considered lower strength than evidence obtained from RCTs or meta-analyses. The three systematic reviews included different studies of antipsychotic medications. Overall, they report positive findings from trials of flupenthixol, clozapine, and fluphenazine, though caution that findings are based on small samples of patients in very few studies. Finally, the systematic reviews report different results related to mood stabilizing medications. Gaynes et al. report no reduction in suicide rates based on one trial of lithium, whereas Mann et al. and NICE report some non-significant reductions in suicide rates for patients receiving lithium.[9-11]

Primary studies included in the current report evaluated antidepressants, atypical antipsychotics, mood stabilizers, and omega-3 supplements and reported their efficacy in prevention of suicidal self-directed violence in civilian populations. Findings from antidepressant trials in civilian populations were consistent with previous reviews on the topic, and did not provide sufficient evidence to make a strong conclusion about the effectiveness of antidepressants in reducing suicides and suicide attempts. We identified nine trials (reported in 10 publications) that evaluated antidepressant medications. Comparisons included various combinations of antidepressant medications versus placebo;[18-23] one antidepressant versus another;[24, 25] antidepressant therapy versus cognitive behavioral therapy (CBT);[23] and antidepressant therapy with and without CBT.[19, 21, 26, 27] Many studies had no suicides in either group. Because of the short duration and low participant numbers, many of these studies would not have had the statistical power and duration of follow-up to allow the medication to effect a change in suicide rates. Therefore, they are felt to be of low strength, and are insufficient for determining the effectiveness of various combinations of antidepressant medications for reducing suicidal self-directed violence.

We found three trials that reported on the effectiveness of quetiapine (1 trial)[28] or adjunctive aripiprazole (2 trials in 3 publications)[29-31] in reducing suicide deaths. These trials were six to eight weeks in duration and none had any suicides reported during the follow-up period. The quetiapine trial reported one suicide attempt in each group (treatment and intervention). Therefore, we concluded there was insufficient evidence to determine antisuicidal benefit. Notably, the previous review by Mann and colleagues reported an antisuicidal effect of clozapine, an atypical antipsychotic medication.[10]

The two trials of mood stabilizers compared lithium versus valproate (2.5 years)[32] and lithium versus citalopram (8 weeks).[33] These trials reported no instances of suicidal self-directed violence for the duration of either study. The previous report by Mann et al., however, found an antisuicidal effect for lithium compared to carbamazepine and amitriptyline.[10] Thus, trials conducted since the Mann et al. report provided insufficient evidence to draw conclusions about the comparative effectiveness of mood stabilizers in preventing suicide attempts. One study conducted outside a country within the scope of this review was suggested for inclusion by reviewers.[34] This study, had it been included in our results, provided insufficient evidence for the effectiveness of lithium in prevention of suicidal self-directed violence when compared to placebo.

Finally, one trial of omega-3 fatty acid supplementation for 12 weeks did not have any suicide deaths in either group.[35]

Psychotherapy Results

Three previously published systematic reviews on this topic all report an overall insufficient to low strength of evidence for the effectiveness of any psychotherapeutic interventions in prevention of self-directed violence.[9-11] In one report (NICE 2011), the authors combined findings from multiple psychotherapy studies with treatment as usual comparison groups, and describe low strength evidence of the effectiveness of these interventions in prevention of self-directed violence.[11] Individual psychotherapy results reported in the three reports include mixed findings related to cognitive therapies, positive findings related to Dialectical Behavior Therapy (DBT) for people with Borderline Personality Disorder, positive findings for interpersonal psychotherapy, null findings for outpatient day hospitalization, positive findings for problem-solving therapy, positive findings for psychoanalytically oriented partial day hospitalization for people with Borderline Personality Disorder, and positive findings for transference-focused psychotherapy. Notably, these results were presented in the previous reports as coming from very few studies with small sample sizes, many methodological flaws, and short-term follow-up assessment periods, suggesting that all findings are of insufficient to low strength and should be interpreted with caution.

All psychotherapy trials meeting criteria for inclusion in this review were sufficiently heterogeneous in terms of type of treatment, duration of treatment, and population characteristics to preclude combination or quantitative comparison. Therefore, psychotherapy trials are grouped for discussion by population: those conducted in patients with Borderline Personality Disorder, recent suicide attempts, a psychotic spectrum disorder, and depression or dysthymia. The strongest evidence (moderate strength) comes from a trial of problem-solving treatment in addition to usual care versus usual care alone for patients with recent suicide attempts.[36] This trial showed no significant benefit of the intervention compared to usual care for the overall group of patients presenting to the hospital after engaging in self-harm behaviors; however, a significant benefit was noted for a sub-population of patients limited to people who had multiple hospitalizations for self-harm prior to the intervention. The other trials of psychotherapy provided insufficient or low strength evidence to draw definitive conclusions, often because of limitations in quality and insufficient statistical power to detect intervention effects on low base-rate outcomes of suicidal self-directed violence.

Three RCTs provided insufficient evidence to draw conclusions about prevention of suicide deaths in populations with Borderline Personality Disorder, largely because no or very few suicides occurred during the trials. One trial showed a significant reduction in suicide attempts with Mentalization Based Treatment (MBT) compared to Structured Clinical Management (SCM),[37] as did a trial comparing DBT with community treatment by experts.[38] Three other studies showed no significant benefit in suicide attempt prevention for Systems Training for Emotional Predictability and Problem Solving (STEPPS) versus treatment as usual,[39] CBT specific to Cluster B personality disorders versus treatment as usual,[40, 41] or DBT versus general psychiatric management.[42]

Few trials reported on prevention of suicide deaths as the outcome of psychotherapy interventions, and of those that did, most were insufficiently powered to detect an effect of the intervention. One study conducted a comparison among people with recent suicide attempts, self-harm incidents, or imminent risk.[43] This trial had several design flaws that contribute to a high potential for bias: non-randomization, baseline differences among the groups, non-blinding, and differing drop-out rates among the groups. Therefore, there was insufficient evidence to draw conclusions about the psychotherapy comparison. Two other studies of people presenting with repeat self-harm reported no suicide events in either treatment or control groups for group therapy,[44] and for intensive case management.[45] Other studies evaluated inventions in similar populations (prior suicide). A study of Attachment-Based Family Therapy versus Enhanced Usual Care showed a reduction in suicide attempts, though design flaws limit the ability to draw a firm conclusion about the results.[46] Likewise, studies comparing Collaborative Assessment and Management of Suicidality (CAMS) versus Enhanced Care As Usual (E-CAU) and skills-based intervention versus a supportive therapy control condition did not use sufficient methodological rigor to enable firm conclusions about effectiveness.[47, 48] Notably, a study of adolescent group therapy compared to routine care resulted in fewer instances of self-harm in the routine care group indicating the possibility of iatrogenic effects in the group treatment condition; however, design flaws in this study preclude the ability to draw firm conclusions based on the results.[49] Finally, one study compared three conditions, CBT, problem-solving therapy, and treatment as usual. This study had few patients and methodological limitations, and therefore provides insufficient evidence related to any of the interventions being investigated.[50]

One study comparing CBT versus supportive counseling in patients with a psychotic spectrum disorder had an unacceptably high risk of bias because therapists were not blinded and delivered both interventions to the participants.[51] Another trial compared the Improving Mood: Promoting Access to Collaborative Treatment (IMPACT) intervention (including a comprehensive depression case management and treatment component) versus usual care in people with depression or dysthymia used methods resulting in an unclear risk of bias.[52] Each of these trials provides insufficient evidence to draw definitive conclusions about the effectiveness of the interventions.

Key Question #3. What is the effectiveness of referral and follow-up services (e.g., strategies designed to provide referrals, improve referral follow-through and attendance, etc.) for reducing rates of suicidal self-directed violence in military and/or Veteran populations?

We did not find any RCTs of suicidal self-directed violence prevention referral and follow-up services in military and/or VA health care settings.

Key Question #4. What lessons can be learned from research on suicidal self-directed violence referral and follow-up services conducted outside of Veteran or military settings that can be applied to Veteran and/or military populations?

The three previously published reports on this topic all report overall insufficient to low strength of evidence for the effectiveness of any referral and follow-up services in prevention of self-directed violence.[9-11] Specific findings from the three reports include positive results from studies on case management/care coordination and 24-hour contact with a mental health professional. Mixed reports of findings came from studies on emergency contact cards and postal contact. Null findings were reported from studies investigating intensive psychosocial follow-up, telephone follow-up, and video education plus family therapy. Notably, these results were presented in the previous reports as coming from very few studies with small sample sizes, many methodological flaws, and short-term follow-up assessment periods, suggesting that all findings are of insufficient to low strength and should be interpreted with caution.

Findings from primary studies included in this report include three studies of postcard interventions to decrease repeated suicidal self-directed violence, which showed mixed results.[53-55] Two studies of Youth-Nominated Support Team (YST) interventions combined with usual care did not significantly reduce risk of suicide attempts or death in suicidal adolescents.[56,57] One study of assertive community treatment compared with community mental health care in difficult-to-engage adults with serious mental illness showed no reduction in suicide deaths or deliberate self-harm incidents.[58] Finally, one trial of a depression care management program resulted in no significant changes in the suicide mortality rate of older adults in primary care settings.[59] However, all these studies were given low strength of evidence ratings and thus limit conclusions about the effectiveness of these interventions.

EVIDENCE REPORT

INTRODUCTION

Suicide is the tenth leading cause of death in the United States (US), with nearly 100 suicides occurring each day and over 36,000 dying by suicide each year.[1] The rate is higher among 25 to 34 year-olds, for whom suicide is the second leading cause of death.[60] While many die by suicide, each suicide represents approximately 25 suicide attempts; the lifetime risk of attempt for the general US population is estimated to be between 1.9 and 8.7 percent.[8, 61] Among Veterans and current military, suicide is a national public health concern. Recent estimates suggest current or former military represent 20 percent of all known suicides in the US,[2] and the rate of suicides among Veterans utilizing Veterans Health Administration (VHA) services is estimated to be higher than the general population.[3] The impact suicide has on family, friends, and community can be overwhelming.[62] Furthermore, suicide attempts may leave the individual severely injured, requiring extensive medical treatment and rehabilitation. The lifetime cost of medical treatment resulting from self-inflicted injuries in 2000 was estimated to be $1 billion.[63] The enormity of the problem has led to several major public health initiatives and a growth in research funding for suicide prevention.[4-7]

Similar to other public health concerns, two main approaches to suicide prevention have taken shape: 1) the identification of individual-level risk factors, with the goal of developing targeted interventions; and 2) the development of population-level prevention strategies. Prior research has identified several risk factors, most notably older age, male sex, physical and mental health disorders (including depression and substance use disorders [SUD]), familial and genetic influences, impulsivity, poor psychosocial support, and access to and knowledge of firearms.[64-67] Unique to the Veteran population are additional risk factors, such as traumatic brain injury (TBI),[68] habituation to violence,[69] and deployment-related issues (strained relationships, stressful events, and post-deployment adjustment).[66, 70] Several autopsy studies of the events leading up to suicide have suggested the majority of individuals who die by suicide exhibit symptoms of depression or other mental health issues prior to death.[71] Additionally, approximately 32 percent of individuals make contact with a mental health care provider and 77 percent make contact with a primary care provider during the year prior to suicide.[72] In one study of Veterans who died by suicide in Oregon, 22 percent made contact with Veteran Affairs (VA) healthcare providers during the year prior to suicide,[73] a rate similar to the estimated one-quarter of Veterans who access VA care annually.[74] As such, targeted interventions have been primarily developed for use in healthcare to treat individuals who present with suicidal thoughts, attempts, or other risk factors, or who are otherwise identified at risk (e.g., as a result of a suicide risk assessment).[75-77] Population-level approaches do not require prior identification of individuals at risk but are designed to reduce suicide using strategies such as providing help-seeking resources (e.g., hotlines, community health centers), environment modification of possible triggers or available means (e.g., media guidelines on suicide reporting, bridge barriers), education and awareness (e.g., public service announcements [PSAs] on the warning signs of suicide), or population-wide screening (e.g., screening all school children).

Despite these and other suicide prevention efforts, the suicide rate in the US has changed relatively little over the past 100 years.[8] The methodological difficulties in studying suicide are similar to those inherent in studying any natural phenomenon (e.g., lack of condition assignment), yet is made more difficult by suicide's relatively low base rate.[60, 78] The paucity of high-quality studies available to offer evidence for effective intervention approaches is not surprising.[10] Furthermore, many suicide risk factors often fail to predict suicide at the individual level, producing numerous false positives.[78] These difficulties highlight the importance of increased focus on research and the continued synthesis of evidence as it is made available, especially with regard to individual-level intervention approaches.

The model below (Figure 1) summarizes the analytical framework used in this report for Veteran, military, and civilian populations. In this report, we focus on individual-level interventions and referral/follow-up services; that is, we focus on interventions and referral/follow-up services that can be implemented with individuals who are identified as being at risk for suicide rather than such interventions that could be implemented with a population of individuals at unknown risk (e.g., large-scale suicide awareness education campaigns). Though the focus of the report is on suicide prevention, we include as outcomes any type of suicidal self-directed violence, defined as, "Behavior that is self-directed and deliberately results in injury or the potential for injury to oneself. There is evidence, whether implicit or explicit, of suicidal intent."[12, 13] We use this terminology throughout this evidence report when possible; however, when describing results from primary studies, we use terminology as reported in the original articles in order to describe outcomes consistent with the primary studies.

Figure 1.   Suicide Prevention Analytical Model

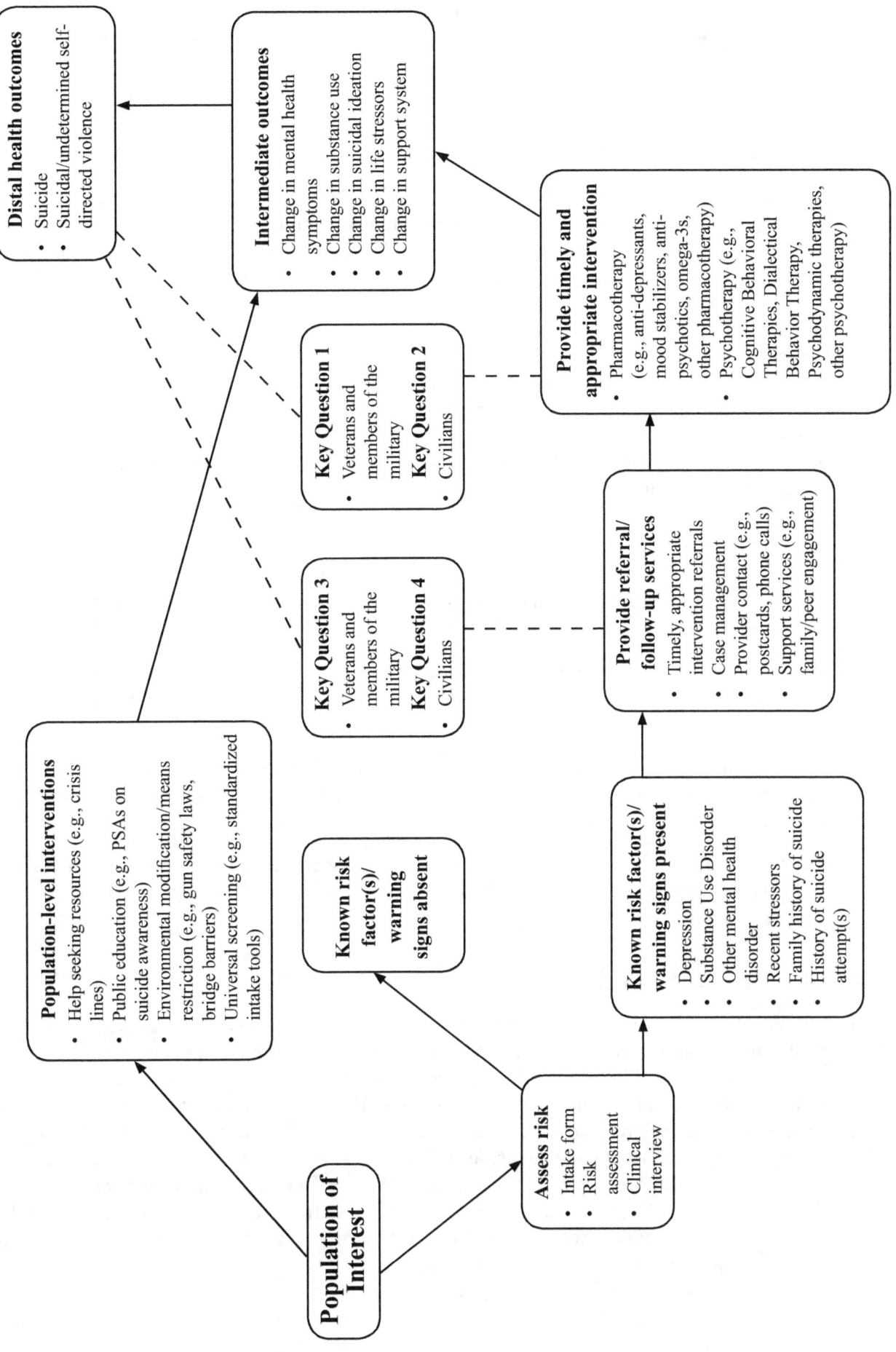

METHODS

TOPIC DEVELOPMENT

This project was requested by the VA/Department of Defense (DoD) Evidence Based Practice Working Group (EBPWG) to support the development of clinical practice guidelines for suicide prevention. The VA/DoD suicide prevention EBPWG requested a systematic review of literature related to suicidal self-directed violence as defined by Crosby et al. and Brenner et al.[12, 13] published since two prior reports on the topic by Mann et al. and Gaynes et al.[9, 10] The workgroup requested a review which was focused on countries and populations of interest due to their similarity to US Veteran and military populations. Though a similar report on self-harm recently conducted by the National Institute for Health and Clinical Excellence (NICE) was released in draft form during the writing of this current report,[11] the EBPWG requested this current ESP report to examine suicidal self-directed violence, specifically, rather than self-harm in general, and to focus on populations most comparable to US Veterans and members of the military. A technical panel comprised of members of this workgroup as well as VA leaders in the field of suicidology provided input.

The final key questions developed a priori in conjunction with the EBPWG are:

Key Question #1. What is the effectiveness of specific interventions for reducing rates of suicidal self-directed violence in military and/or Veteran populations?

Key Question #2. What lessons can be learned from suicidal self-directed violence prevention intervention research conducted outside of Veteran or military settings that can be applied to Veteran and/or military populations?

Key Question #3. What is the effectiveness of referral and follow-up services (e.g., strategies designed to provide referrals, improve referral follow-through and attendance, etc.) for reducing rates of suicidal self-directed violence in military and/or Veteran populations?

Key Question #4. What lessons can be learned from research on suicidal self-directed violence referral and follow-up services conducted outside of Veteran or military settings that can be applied to Veteran and/or military populations?

SEARCH STRATEGY

The VA/DoD suicide prevention EBPWG workgroup requested a systematic review of literature related to suicidal self-directed violence published since two prior reports on the topic by Mann et al. and Gaynes et al.[9, 10] The workgroup requested a review which was focused on countries and populations of interest due to their similarity to US Veteran and military populations. Though a previous systematic review was conducted by Shekelle and colleagues in 2009,[14] the EBPWG requested that the current review include studies of pharmacotherapy and psychotherapy interventions, which were largely excluded from this previous report; and, therefore, we used the end search date from the Mann et al. review as the starting point for the current search. To identify relevant systematic reviews and controlled trials, we searched PubMed, PsycINFO, the

Cochrane Database of Systematic Reviews®, and the Cochrane Central Register of Controlled Trials®. Our search focused on identifying all new studies published since the systematic reviews completed by Mann et al. in 2005 and Gaynes et al. in 2004,[9, 10] and covered the period from January 2005 to November 18, 2011. Therefore, we used a similar search strategy including suicide and all related terms; we also included interventions and military and Veteran populations as search terms (Appendix A). We limited the search to peer-reviewed articles involving human subjects and published in the English language that were not included in previously published systematic reviews on the topic.[9, 10]

To assure that our search did not miss relevant articles on suicidal self-directed violence interventions, we obtained additional articles from systematic reviews, reference lists of pertinent studies, reviews, editorials, and consulting experts. Additionally, though the focus of the requested review was on interventions and services to reduce suicide, we included any intervention reporting on suicidal self-directed violence as an outcome to include as comprehensive a list of articles as possible with the potential for suicidal self-directed violence prevention efficacy.

STUDY SELECTION

Titles and abstracts were reviewed by doctoral level investigators and project research associates trained in the critical analysis of literature. Eligibility of full-text articles was initially carefully ascertained by one reviewer and the accuracy of all assessments was then checked by a second reviewer. All disagreements were resolved by consensus.

To determine the evidence base for interventions and referral/follow-up services to prevent suicide in Veteran and military populations, we examined randomized controlled trials (RCTs) of interventions and referral/follow-up services that can be implemented at an individual level for a person identified as being at risk for suicide. Though observational studies and studies lacking a control or comparison condition can provide important information about the natural course of suicide, the focus of this report was on RCTs in an attempt to examine the highest quality evidence with the least potential for biased results.

Our review was designed to detect the highest quality evidence evaluating individual-level interventions and study settings/populations that most closely approximate US Veteran and military populations. Therefore, though we used selection criteria similar to those used in the reviews by Mann et al. and Gaynes et al., our review differs from these reviews in: 1) excluding observational studies, 2) excluding trials of community-based interventions, and 3) excluding trials conducted in countries dissimilar to the US.

We classified studies as pharmacotherapy interventions, psychotherapy interventions, or referral and follow-up services. We defined interventions as treatments designed to impact a condition, symptom, or behavior. Referral and follow-up services were any services that were provided to patients that were primarily designed to facilitate access to interventions rather than treat a condition, symptom, or behavior. Because many interventions include components designed to increase adherence and attendance, we classified any study describing an intervention component as an "intervention" study rather than a "referral and follow-up services" study even if it also included components of referral and follow-up services. Therefore, the studies designated as referral and follow-up services were described by the authors as solely designed to increase access to, attendance at, and/or adherence to other interventions not included in the study design.

Below are listed the specific inclusion criteria used to select studies for each Key Question, respectively:

Key Question #1 – Primary literature review of studies published between 2005 and November 18, 2011, with the following characteristics:

- Population: Any Veteran and/or military patient subgroup from the US, United Kingdom (UK), Canada, New Zealand, and Australia.

- Intervention: Any intervention with the potential to reduce or prevent suicidal self-directed violence including interventions related to environmental modification, psychotherapy, medication, somatic treatment, and monitoring. This report will include individual-level interventions applicable to clinical encounter settings (i.e., services that can be provided to individual patients). This report will exclude more broadly focused population-level or public health types of interventions designed to be implemented with large groups of people with unknown individual suicide risk levels.

- Comparator: No intention to limit by comparator.

- Outcomes: Suicidal self-directed violence including suicide attempt and suicide, not including self-directed violence ideation and undetermined or non-suicidal self-directed violence (i.e., behavior resulting in injury for which there is *unclear or no implicit or explicit evidence of intent to die*).

- Timing: Any length of follow-up.

- Setting: US Veteran or military inpatient or outpatient settings.

Key Question #2 – Review of suicidal self-directed violence prevention intervention research conducted in non-Veteran and/or non-military settings with the same parameters as Key Question #1 other than population.

Key Question #3 – Primary literature review of studies published between 2005 and November 18, 2011, with the following characteristics:

- Population: Any Veteran and/or military patient subgroup from the US, UK, Canada, New Zealand, and Australia.

- Intervention: Any referral or follow-up service with the potential to reduce or prevent suicidal self-directed violence including referral/follow-up services related to care coordination, provider contact, and social support. This report will include individual-level referral/follow-up services applicable to clinical encounter settings (i.e., services that can be provided to individual patients). This report will exclude more broadly focused population-level or public health types of referral/follow-up services designed to be implemented with large groups of people with unknown individual suicide risk levels.

- Comparator: No intention to limit by comparator.

- Outcomes: Suicidal self-directed violence including suicide attempt and suicide, not including self-directed violence ideation and undetermined or non-suicidal self-directed violence (i.e., behavior resulting in injury for which there is *unclear or no implicit or explicit evidence of intent to die*).

- Timing: Any length of follow-up.

- Setting: Any non-Veteran or non-military inpatient or outpatient setting.

Key Question #4 – Review of suicidal self-directed violence referral and follow-up services research conducted in non-Veteran and/or non-military settings with the same parameters as Key Question #3 other than population.

The complete study selection form including abstract and full-text codes is included in Appendix B.

DATA ABSTRACTION

For controlled trials, we abstracted information on setting, population characteristics, interventions, comparators, number of subjects, length of follow-up, outcome assessment methods, and results. For systematic reviews, we abstracted information on time period and databases searched and eligibility criteria used; and for all included studies that also met our eligibility criteria, we also abstracted information on study designs, setting, sample size, population characteristics, interventions and comparators, and main results.

QUALITY ASSESSMENT

We assessed the quality of systematic reviews using predefined criteria established by Oxman and Guyatt in 1991.[15] The Oxman and Guyatt quality rating system consists of nine questions that involve assessing the adequacy of systematic review methods including searching, reporting of inclusion criteria, study selection, validity assessment, data synthesis, and conclusions. Each question is scored as 'Yes,' 'Partially/Can't Tell,' or 'No'. The overall quality is scored based on a scale of 1 to 7, where 1 represents the presence of extensive flaws and 7 represents the presence of minimal flaws (Appendix C).

We assessed the risk of bias of controlled trials using the tool described in version 5.1.0 of the *Cochrane Handbook for Systematic Reviews of Interventions*.[16] The Cochrane Collaboration's tool for assessing risk of bias involves assessing the adequacy of the following six domains: sequence generation, allocation concealment, blinding of participants, personnel and outcome assessors, handling of incomplete data, selective outcome reporting, and any other sources of bias. Adequacy for each domain is rated as 'yes,' 'no,' or 'unclear'. The overall risk of bias for each controlled trial is then rated as 'low,' 'unclear,' or 'high' based on the reviewer's judgment of the plausibility that the biases have seriously weakened their confidence in the results (Appendix D).

Two reviewers independently assessed the quality of each study. Reviewers then compared their ratings and resolved all differences through discussion or by consulting a third party when consensus could not be reached.

We assessed studies for applicability to US Veterans and members of the US Armed Forces, and included a qualitative assessment of applicability to these populations of interest in the discussion section of this report.

DATA SYNTHESIS

We constructed evidence tables showing the study characteristics and results for all included studies, organized by key question, intervention, or clinical condition, as appropriate. We critically analyzed studies to compare their characteristics, methods, and findings. We compiled a summary of findings for each key question or clinical topic, and drew conclusions based on qualitative synthesis of the findings.

We also report findings as described in the prior systematic review by Mann et al. Because our review was designed to be an update to the report by Mann et al., we have not re-evaluated the source studies included in their report.

RATING THE BODY OF EVIDENCE

We assessed the overall quality of evidence for outcomes based on the guidance established for the Evidence-based Practice Center (EPC) Program of the Agency for Healthcare Research and Quality (AHRQ) (Appendix E).[17] The AHRQ EPC approach requires assessment of four key domains: risk of bias, consistency, directness, and precision. When relevant, reviewers may also consider the following additional optional domains: dose-response association, plausible confounding that would decrease the observed effect, strength of association (magnitude of effect), and publication bias. Ratings across the multiple domains are then combined to formulate a global assessment of the overall strength of the evidence. The strength of the evidence level is rated as 'high,' 'moderate,' 'low,' or 'insufficient' based on the reviewers' confidence that the evidence reflects the true effect and their judgment about the likelihood that further research will change the estimate.

Our review was designed only to examine studies published since June, 2005, so we consider the findings from the Mann et al. review to assess the contributions of pre-2005 literature on the overall strength of evidence. However, because Mann et al. used different quality assessment and data synthesis methodology, the combination of results from the two reports should be interpreted with caution.

To provide a summary of evidence combining the results of the Mann et al. and our reviews, we report all positive findings from the Mann et al. review along with results from the studies included in our review. We did not present negative findings from the Mann et al. report because it was impossible to discern whether these results represented a lack of good quality evidence or a true negative result. Acknowledging the limitations in combining studies from two reviews in this way, we have clearly identified those studies from the Mann review separately from the newer studies included in our review.

PEER REVIEW

A draft version of this report was reviewed by eight technical experts, as well as clinical leadership. Their comments and our responses are presented in Appendix AA.

RESULTS

LITERATURE FLOW

We reviewed 16,426 titles and abstracts from the electronic search, and an additional 92 from reference mining for a total of 16,518 references. After applying inclusion/exclusion criteria at the abstract level, 16,110 references were excluded. We retrieved 408 full-text articles for further review and another 336 references were excluded. We identified a total of 85 references for inclusion in the current review, including 38 RCTs (reported in 47 publications) and 23 systematic reviews (reported in 25 publications). We grouped the studies by key question, type of intervention, route of administration, and clinical condition. Figure 2 details the number of references related to exclusion criteria and publication type.

Figure 2. Literature Flow Chart[a]

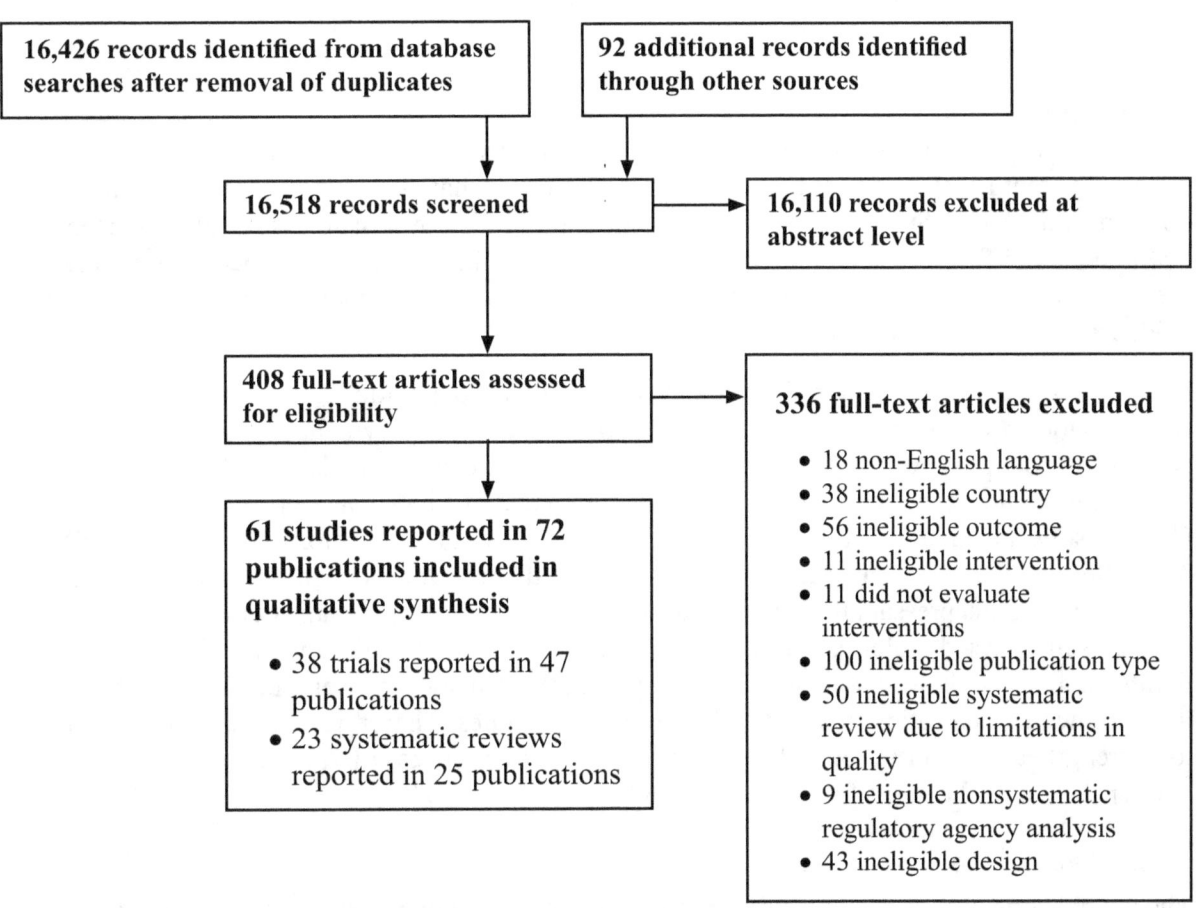

[a] Modified from the PRISMA flow diagram.[79]

KEY QUESTION #1. What is the effectiveness of specific interventions for reducing rates of suicidal self-directed violence in military and/or Veteran populations?

We did not find any RCTs of suicidal self-directed violence prevention interventions in military and/or VA health care settings.

KEY QUESTION #2. What lessons can be learned from self-directed violence prevention intervention research conducted outside of VA or military settings that can be applied to Veteran and/or military populations?

Pharmacotherapy Interventions

Summary of Findings

Antidepressants

The conclusions of three systematic reviews with similar key questions to the current report were consistent in relation to antidepressants.[9-11] All found that available evidence from trials does not show a benefit for reducing suicide, but caution that rates of suicide may have been too low to detect differences. Although observational studies show a correlation between increasing prescription rates and decreasing suicide rates, this evidence is considered lower strength than evidence obtained from RCTs or meta-analyses.

Findings from antidepressant trials in non-Veteran/military populations were consistent with previous reviews on the topic, and did not provide sufficient evidence to make a strong conclusion about the effectiveness of antidepressants in reducing suicidal self-directed violence. We identified nine trials (reported in 10 publications) that evaluated antidepressant medications. Comparisons included various combinations of antidepressant medications versus placebo;[18-23] one antidepressant versus another;[24, 25] antidepressant therapy versus cognitive behavioral therapy (CBT);[23] and antidepressant therapy with and without CBT.[19, 21, 26, 27] Many studies reported no suicidal self-directed violence in either group. Because of the short duration and low participant numbers, many of these studies would not have had the statistical power and duration of follow-up to allow the medication to affect a change in suicide rates. Therefore, they are felt to be of low strength, and are insufficient for determining the effectiveness of various combinations of antidepressant medications for reducing suicides.

Atypical Antipsychotics

The conclusions of three systematic reviews with similar key questions to the current report were consistent in relation to atypical antipsychotic medications.[9-11] The three reports included different studies of antipsychotic medications. Overall, they report positive findings from trials of flupenthixol, clozapine, and fluphenazine, though caution that findings are based on small samples of patients in very few studies.

We found three trials that reported on the effectiveness of quetiapine (1 trial)[28] or adjunctive aripiprazole (2 trials in 3 publications)[29-31] in reducing suicide deaths. These trials were six to eight weeks in duration and none had any suicides reported during the follow-up period. The quetiapine trial reported one suicide attempt in each group (treatment and intervention). Therefore, we concluded there was insufficient evidence to determine antisuicidal benefit. Notably, the Mann et al. review found an antisuicidal effect of clozapine, an atypical antipsychotic medication.[10]

Mood Stabilizers

The conclusions of three systematic reviews with similar key questions to the current report were consistent in relation to atypical mood stabilizers.[9-11] The three reports included different studies of mood stabilizers. The systematic reviews report different results related to mood stabilizing medications. Gaynes et al. report no reduction in suicide rates based on one trial of lithium, whereas Mann et al. and NICE report some non-significant reductions in suicide rates for patients receiving lithium.[9-11]

The two trials of mood stabilizers compared lithium versus valproate (2.5 years)[32] and lithium versus citalopram (8 weeks).[33] These trials did not report any occurrences of suicidal self-directed violence during the course of the trials. The Mann et al. review found an antisuicidal effect for lithium compared to carbamazepine and amitriptyline in trials published prior to June, 2005.[10] Thus, these trials provided insufficient evidence to draw conclusions about the comparative effectiveness of mood stabilizers in preventing suicidal self-directed violence.

One study conducted in a country outside the scope of this review was suggested for inclusion by reviewers.[34] This study, had it been included in our results, provided insufficient evidence for the effectiveness of lithium in prevention of suicidal self-directed violence when compared to placebo.

Omega-3 Fatty Acid Supplementation

One trial of omega-3 fatty acid supplementation for 12 weeks did not have any suicide deaths in either group.[35]

Studies of Efficacy

Systematic Reviews

We identified 20 new relevant systematic reviews (in 22 publications) that had been published subsequent to Mann et al.[10, 80-101] However, the utility of the conclusions from these systematic reviews was limited due to scope differences. Specifically, in all cases for our outcomes of interest (i.e., suicidal self-directed violence), conclusions from existing new reviews were based on groups of primary studies with a broader range of designs (i.e., observational), publication dates (i.e., before 2005) and from a broader range of countries than our focus of the US, United Kingdom, Canada, New Zealand, and Australia. Therefore, we were only able to use existing new reviews as an additional source of identifying new primary RCTs. Appendices F and G document the quality assessment of the systematic reviews found in our search, as well as data from the RCTs included in the reviews.

We found three systematic reviews that addressed key questions that are similar to those addressed in this report,[9-11] and a summary of findings from these reports are included in

Appendix H. Overall, these three systematic reviews report that all findings are based on few studies with limited sample sizes, some methodological quality concerns, and short term follow-up assessment periods; therefore, pharmacotherapy findings should be interpreted with caution. The findings from the Mann et al. report, which was conducted with a similar search strategy to this report with non-overlapping search dates, are combined with the results from our search and presented in the following results section and associated tables.

Randomized Controlled Trials (RCTs)

The majority of trials focused on patients with depression, but half specifically excluded those who posed a suicidal risk. The majority of trials did not involve the necessary sample sizes (mean, 284.4 patients; standard deviation, 177.8) or follow-up durations (median, 8 weeks; range, 4 weeks to 2.5 years) required to adequately evaluate risk of suicide attempts or suicides. Therefore, these trials generally provided inadequate to low strength evidence for drawing conclusions about risk of suicide attempts and suicides. Data abstraction, risk of bias assessment, and strength of evidence rating tables are included in Appendices J through L.

We also report a summary of sample sizes, outcome definitions and results from all RCTs included in this review, along with a description of the purpose of the study in order to examine possible relationships among study intent, design and outcome. Of particular interest was whether studies which were designed to treat suicidal self-directed violence might be better powered to detect effects of such a low base rate outcome when compared to studies designed to treat another related but more common outcome such as depression. These results are presented in Appendix I for studies investigating pharmacotherapy interventions. Notably, there does not appear to be a strong relationship between sample size (and, by extension, statistical power) and whether or not the studies were reportedly designed to treat suicidal self-directed violence versus other outcomes.

Antidepressants

The conclusions of the Mann et al., Gaynes et al., and NICE reports were similar in relation to antidepressants.[9-11] All found that available evidence from trials does not show a benefit for reducing suicide, but caution that rates of suicide may have been too low to detect differences. Although observational studies show a correlation between increasing prescription rates and decreasing suicide rates, this evidence is considered lower strength than evidence obtained from RCTs or meta-analyses.

Antidepressants versus Placebo. The Mann review found that antidepressants were not associated with a benefit over placebo for suicidal self-directed violence.[10]

The majority of the RCTs published subsequent to the Mann review provided insufficient evidence for drawing conclusions about associations between antidepressants and suicidal self-directed violence.[18-22] The strength of this evidence was limited both by trials that apparently did not assess suicide deaths[18, 20] and those that did, in which small sample sizes and/or inadequate follow-up durations likely led to a lack of observed events.[19, 21, 22] The only trial that reported any suicide deaths had low potential for bias, but still provided low strength evidence of no significant difference between paroxetine 38.8 mg (mean) and placebo in suicide deaths at week eight among 180 civilian adults with moderate to severe depression (0.8% compared with 0, P not reported).[23]

RCTs published subsequent to the Mann review also provided low strength evidence of no significant difference between escitalopram 13.2 mg (mean),[20] fluoxetine 32.8 mg (mean maximal),[19, 21] or paroxetine 10 mg[18] compared with placebo in suicide attempts in depressed children and adolescents.

Antidepressants versus Antidepressants. We included two RCTs that directly compared different antidepressant medication regimens.[24, 25] These trials provided insufficient evidence to draw conclusions about differential effects on risk of suicide death due to insufficient statistical power and a lack of observed events. However, one trial with an unclear risk of bias provided low strength evidence that escitalopram, taken in combination with (0 events) or without bupropion sustained-release (0 events), significantly reduced risk of suicide attempts at seven months compared with venlafaxine extended release plus mirtazapine (2.3%, $P=0.0162$) when taken in civilian adults with either recurrent or chronic major depressive disorder.[25]

Antidepressants Alone versus Antidepressants plus CBT. We included three RCTs with unclear risk of bias that compared antidepressants alone versus antidepressants plus CBT in adolescents with major depressive disorder.[19, 21, 26, 27] These trials provided insufficient evidence to draw conclusions about prevention of suicide deaths as only one trial reported assessment of suicide deaths, and there were no observed events for fluoxetine alone or fluoxetine plus CBT after 36 weeks in 216 adolescents with major depressive disorder.[19, 21] Additionally, compared to taking antidepressants alone, these trials provided low strength evidence that combination treatment with CBT plus antidepressants did not significantly improve protective effects against suicidal self-injury adverse events at 12 weeks,[26] suicidal acts at 28 weeks,[27] or suicide attempts at 36 weeks.[19, 21] In one of these trials,[26] subgroup analyses found that participants with higher than median baseline suicidal ideation were more likely to experience a self-harm event (suicidal or non-suicidal) if they were treated with venlafaxine than with a Selective Serotonin Reuptake Inhibitor (SSRI), and participants who received a benzodiazepine in addition to an antidepressant were more likely to experience suicidal self-injury adverse events.

Antidepressants versus CBT. We included one RCT with an unclear risk of bias that provided low-strength evidence of no significant difference between paroxetine 38.8 mg (mean) and cognitive therapy in suicide deaths at week eight among 180 civilian adults with moderate to severe depression (0.8% compared with 0, P not reported).[23]

Atypical Antipsychotics

The Mann et al., Gaynes et al., and NICE reports included different studies of antipsychotic medications.[9-11] Overall, they report positive findings from trials of flupenthixol, clozapine, and fluphenazine, though caution that findings are based on small samples of patients in very few studies. The Mann review found an antisuicidal effect for clozapine in two randomized, controlled trials in adults with schizophrenia spectrum disorders.[10] These findings are summarized in the strength of evidence tables provided in Appendix L and provide insufficient to low strength evidence for the suicidal self-directed violence preventive effect of clozapine for adults with schizophrenia spectrum disorders.

Trials of quetiapine[28] and aripiprazole[29-31] published subsequent to the Mann review did not detect benefit for suicide prevention in civilians with mood disorders. In fact, no suicides occurred in any of the three trials. This is likely because these trials: 1) enrolled lower-risk patients who would be expected to have a low base rate of suicide (protocols specified exclusion of patients that posed a suicidal risk); 2) involved inadequate follow-up durations to detect such a low base rate of suicide (6-8 weeks); and 3) had relatively small treatment group sample sizes that were likely underpowered to detect a low base rate of suicide (range, 176 to 191 patients).

Risk of bias was low in the placebo-controlled trial of quetiapine monotherapy (300 or 600 mg) in 542 outpatients with bipolar depression.[28] During the eight-week trial, only two patients attempted suicide (1 in each of the quetiapine groups) and there were no suicides. Risk of bias was unclear in the two identically-designed, placebo-controlled trials of aripiprazole (mean dose range, 11.0 mg/day to 11.8 mg/day) as adjunctive treatment to standard antidepressant therapy in the treatment of 743 patients with major depressive disorder who have shown an incomplete response to the same antidepressant therapy.[29-31] There were no suicides during the six-week treatment periods in either trial.

Mood Stabilizers

The Mann review found an antisuicidal effect for lithium compared to carbamazepine and amitriptyline in a long-term (2.5 years) randomized, controlled trial of 378 German adults with affective disorders, providing insufficient to low strength evidence for the suicidal self-directed violence preventive effect of lithium for adults with affective disorders. [10]

However, two RCTs of lithium published subsequent to the Mann review did not detect benefit for suicide prevention in civilians with mood disorders.[32, 33] There was no significant difference between lithium 0.6–1.0 mEq/dl and valproate 45–125 µg/ml detected over 2.5 years in 98 civilian bipolar patients in a major depressive or mixed episode who had a past suicide attempt.[32] There were no suicide deaths and no significant difference between lithium and valproate in suicide attempts (12% compared with 16%; *P*-value not reported) or in time to suicide attempt (log-rank test). Risk of bias was unclear in this trial due to insufficient information to permit firm judgments for the majority of the bias domains. Our uncertainty about the impact of the incomplete outcome data raised the most doubt about the results of this trial. The loss to follow-up was 26 percent and somewhat higher in the lithium group (31% compared with 20%), and those lost to follow-up had more previous psychiatric hospitalizations and were more likely to report a history of childhood abuse. However, since neither of those potential risk factors has strong empirical evidence of association with suicide attempts or death and we are also uncertain whether the proportion of missing data is enough to induce a clinically relevant bias in effect size, we have fair confidence in the trial's results.

In an RCT with low potential for bias, there were no suicide deaths or attempts at four weeks with citalopram 20 mg once daily, taken with or without lithium 300 mg, in 80 severely depressed, civilian adults.[33]

Although both trials enrolled high-risk participants and the 2.5-year follow-up period used in one of the trials was sufficiently long to capture suicide outcomes,[32] neither trial was adequately powered to detect differences in suicide attempts or deaths.

Finally, one study conducted in the countries outside the scope of this review was suggested for inclusion by reviewers.[34] This study, had it been included in our results, was judged to have a high risk of bias due to having a high loss to follow-up, baseline differences between groups, and other factors. The trial compared lithium to placebo, resulting in a suicide death rate of 0/84 (0%) in the intervention group and 3/83 (3.6%) in the control group, though these differences were not statistically significant; the combined sample size was 167. The authors report similar results between the two groups in terms of suicide attempts. Overall, the results from this study provide insufficient evidence for the effectiveness of lithium in prevention of suicidal self-directed violence when compared to placebo.

Omega-3 Fatty Acid Supplementation

Evidence is insufficient to draw conclusions about the antisuicidal effects of omega-3 fatty acid supplementation.[35] In an RCT with low potential for bias, there were no suicide deaths at 12 weeks with eicosapentaenoic acid 1.2 mg plus docosahexaenoic acid 0.9 mg or placebo in 49 civilian adults who presented to an academic teaching hospital in Dublin, Ireland after an act of repeat self-harm.

Psychotherapy Interventions

Summary of Findings

All psychotherapy trials meeting criteria for inclusion in this review were sufficiently heterogeneous in terms of type of treatment, duration of treatment, and population characteristics to preclude combination or quantitative comparison. Therefore, psychotherapy trials are grouped for discussions by population: those conducted in patients with Borderline Personality Disorder, recent suicide attempts, a psychotic spectrum disorder, and depression or dysthymia.

Three previously published systematic reviews on this topic all report overall insufficient to low strength of evidence for the effectiveness of any psychotherapeutic interventions in the prevention of self-directed violence.[9-11] The authors of these reviews describe these limitations as being due to basing findings on very few studies with limited sample sizes, some methodological quality concerns, and short term follow-up assessment periods, as well as difficulties studying such low base-rate outcomes.

Psychotherapy Interventions for People with Borderline Personality Disorder

Psychotherapy results reported in the Mann et al. systematic review included insufficient to low strength evidence supporting the suicidal self-directed violence preventive effects of Dialectical Behavior Therapy (DBT) and psychoanalytically oriented partial day hospitalization for people with Borderline Personality Disorder.

Three RCTs provided insufficient evidence to draw conclusions about prevention of suicide deaths in populations with Borderline Personality Disorder, largely because no or very few suicides occurred during the trials. One trial showed a significant reduction in suicide attempts with Mentalization Based Treatment (MBT) compared to Structured Clinical Management (SCM),[37] as did a trial comparing DBT with community treatment by experts.[38] Three other studies showed no significant benefit in suicide attempt prevention for Systems Training for Emotional Predictability and Problem Solving (STEPPS) versus treatment as usual,[39] CBT specific to Cluster B personality disorders versus treatment as usual,[40, 41] or DBT versus general psychiatric management.[42]

*Psychotherapy Interventions for People with Recent Suicide Attempts, Recent Self-Harm
Incidents, or Imminent Risk*

Psychotherapy results reported in the Mann et al. systematic review included insufficient to low
strength evidence supporting the suicidal self-directed violence preventive effects of cognitive
therapies, cognitive therapy, interpersonal psychotherapy, and problem-solving therapy.

The strongest evidence (moderate strength) obtained from primary studies included in this
report comes from a trial of problem-solving therapy in addition to usual care versus usual care
alone for patients with recent suicide attempts.[36] This trial showed no significant benefit of the
intervention compared to usual care when examining a patient population of people hospitalized
for a wide variety of self-harming behaviors; patients participating in DBT were excluded from
the study. The authors report examination of an a priori hypothesis to see whether there were
different treatment effects for patients whose index hospitalization was the first time they were
hospitalized for self-harm behavior versus patients who were repeatedly hospitalized for self-
harm behavior prior to the intervention. They report that the treatment showed no significant
effect in patients who were hospitalized for the first time; however, there were significantly fewer
re-presentations to the hospital for self-harm behaviors for both consenting and all (consenting
and non-consenting, i.e., intention-to-treat [ITT] analysis) patients when only patients who had
repeated hospitalizations for self-harm prior to the intervention were considered. There were
also significantly fewer participants who self-reported engaging in self-harm behaviors from the
group of consenting patients when only patients who had repeated hospitalizations for self-harm
prior to the intervention were considered, though this self-report data was not able to be obtained
from non-consenting patients for the ITT analysis. The authors report that analyses adjusting for
treatment location and therapist nesting had no effect on the results. Finally, a similar pattern of
statistically significant results for patient groups was reported for time to re-presentation to the
hospital for self-harm behaviors, with patients hospitalized for repeat self-harm in the treatment
group showing a significant improvement in time to re-presentation when compared to patients
in the control condition; these results were significant for both consenting patients as well as the
combined group of consenting and non-consenting patients (i.e., the ITT analysis).

Few trials reported on prevention of suicide deaths as the outcome of psychotherapy
interventions, and of those that did, most were insufficiently powered to detect an effect of the
intervention. One study conducted a comparison among people with recent suicide attempts,
self-harm incidents, or imminent risk.[43] This trial had several design flaws that contribute to a
high potential for bias: non-randomization, baseline differences among the groups, non-blinding,
and differing drop-out rates among the groups. Therefore, there was insufficient evidence to
draw conclusions about the psychotherapy comparison. Two other studies of people presenting
with repeat self-harm reported no suicide events in either treatment or control groups for
group therapy,[44] and for intensive case management.[45] Other studies evaluated inventions in
similar populations (prior suicidal self-directed violence). A study of Attachment-Based Family
Therapy versus Enhanced Usual Care showed a reduction in suicide attempts, though design
flaws limit the ability to draw a firm conclusion about the results.[46] Likewise, studies comparing
Collaborative Assessment and Management of Suicidality (CAMS) versus Enhanced Care As
Usual (E-CAU) and skills-based intervention versus a supportive therapy control condition
did not use sufficient methodological rigor to enable firm conclusions about effectiveness.[47,48]

Notably, a study of adolescent group therapy compared to routine care resulted in fewer instances of self-harm in the routine care group indicating the possibility of iatrogenic effects in the group treatment condition; however, design flaws in this study preclude the ability to draw firm conclusions based on the results.[49] Finally, one study compared three conditions: CBT, problem-solving therapy, and treatment as usual. This study had few patients and methodological limitations and, therefore, provides insufficient evidence related to any of the interventions being investigated.[50]

Psychotherapy Interventions for People with a Psychotic Spectrum Disorder

One study comparing CBT versus supportive counseling in patients with a psychotic spectrum disorder had an unacceptably high risk of bias because therapists were not blinded and delivered both interventions to the participants.[51] This trial provided insufficient evidence to draw definitive conclusions about the effectiveness of the intervention.

Psychotherapy Interventions for People with a Depression or Dysthymia

One trial comparing the Improving Mood: Promoting Access to Collaborative Treatment (IMPACT) intervention (including a comprehensive depression case management and treatment component) versus usual care in people with depression or dysthymia had methods that suggested an unclear risk of bias.[52] This trial provided insufficient evidence to draw definitive conclusions about the effectiveness of the intervention.

Studies of Efficacy

Systematic Reviews

Our search identified 24 new systematic reviews relevant to psychotherapy published in 25 articles subsequent to Mann 2005.[14, 86, 87, 89, 90, 93, 94, 96, 98, 100, 102-116] Of these, 13 were rated high quality according to the Oxman and Guyatt validation index[15] and are included in the summary below.[14, 87, 98, 102, 104, 106, 107, 109, 111-115] Eleven were rated lower quality and are not discussed further in this report.

Of the 13 high quality systematic reviews, most included only primary studies that were outside the scope of this review: primary studies with a broader range of study designs (i.e., observational studies); publication dates (i.e., before 2005); and from a broader range of countries than our focus on the US, United Kingdom, Canada, New Zealand, and Australia. Of the potentially eligible RCTs identified from the high quality systematic reviews, only one contributed relevant data related to psychotherapeutic interventions and is included in our review of primary studies.[52] Appendices M and N summarize quality assessment and data abstraction from the included systematic reviews.

In addition to these reviews, we included and summarized findings from three other systematic reviews with similar key questions to this current report. These three previously published reports on this topic all report findings of psychotherapeutic interventions with different combinations of studies into categories, making comparisons across reports difficult.[9-11] Results are reported in Appendix S, and all three reports note the overall insufficient to low strength of evidence for the effectiveness of any psychotherapeutic interventions in prevention of self-directed violence. The authors of the other reviews describe these limitations as being due to basing findings on very few studies with limited sample sizes, some methodological quality concerns, and short term follow-up assessment periods, as well as difficulties studying such low base-rate outcomes. Overall, combination of findings from multiple psychotherapy studies compared to treatment as usual resulted in low strength evidence of the effectiveness of these interventions in prevention of self-directed violence. Individual psychotherapy results included mixed findings related to cognitive therapies, positive findings related to DBT for people with Borderline Personality Disorder, positive findings for interpersonal psychotherapy, null findings for outpatient day hospitalization, positive findings for problem-solving therapy, positive findings for psychoanalytically oriented partial day hospitalization for people with Borderline Personality Disorder, and positive findings for transference-focused psychotherapy. Notably, these results were presented in the previous reports as coming from very few studies with small sample sizes, many methodological flaws, and short-term follow-up assessment periods, suggesting that all findings are of insufficient to low strength and should be interpreted with caution. The findings from the Mann et al. report, which was conducted with a similar search strategy to this report with non-overlapping search dates, are combined with the results from our search and presented in the following results section and associated tables.

Randomized Controlled Trials (RCTs)

Appendices Q through S summarize quality assessment, risk of bias, and strength of evidence ratings from the included primary studies.

We also report a summary of sample sizes, outcome definitions, and results from all RCTs included in this review along with a description of the purpose of the study in order to examine possible relationships among study intent and design, and outcome. Of particular interest was whether studies which were designed to treat suicidal self-directed violence might be better powered to detect effects of such a low base rate outcome when compared to studies designed to treat another related but more common outcome such as depression. These results are presented in Appendix O for studies investigating psychotherapy interventions. Notably, there does not appear to be a strong relationship between sample size (and, by extension, statistical power) and whether or not the studies were reportedly designed to treat suicidal self-directed violence versus other outcomes.

Psychotherapy Interventions for People with Borderline Personality Disorder

The Mann review found that both psychoanalytically-oriented partial hospitalization and DBT reduced suicidal self-directed violence compared with standard after care.[10] Notably, these results were presented in the Mann et al. report as coming from very few studies with small sample sizes, methodological flaws, and short-term follow-up assessment periods, suggesting that these findings should be interpreted with caution. Overall, these studies provide insufficient to low strength evidence for the effectiveness of the interventions.

Evidence published since the Mann review included six trials investigating the relative effectiveness of interventions for the treatment of Borderline Personality Disorder in reducing suicidal self-directed violence. Due to the heterogeneity of study populations and interventions, the evidence from each study is reported separately. Detailed descriptions of the various interventions are contained in the data abstraction tables (Appendix Q).

Two studies (Bateman et al., 2008 and Bateman et al., 2009) examined MBT, though the former compared this treatment to treatment as usual, and the latter used SCM as the control condition.[37, 117] Compared to SCM, there is low-strength evidence that MBT significantly reduced the proportion of patients with life-threatening suicide attempts after 18 months (2.8% compared with 25.4%; effect size of d = .65) and those with severe self-harm incidents (23.9% compared with 42.9%; effect size of d = .62).[37] However, the trial that compared MBT with SCM provided insufficient evidence to draw conclusions about their relative effectiveness in self-directed violence prevention due to the presence of an unacceptably high risk of bias, as well as imprecise data.[117]

Blum and colleagues (2008) conducted an RCT of STEPPS versus treatment as usual.[39] This trial provides low-strength evidence of no significant between-group differences in time to first suicide attempt and time to first self-harm incidents.

Two articles (Davidson et al., 2006 and Davidson et al., 2010) describe an RCT of CBT specific to Cluster B personality disorders versus treatment as usual.[40, 41] This trial of 106 participants provides low-strength evidence that there is a non-significant effect of the intervention on number of subjects with suicidal acts over six years (56% compared with 73%; Odds ratio [OR] 0.37; 95% Confidence Interval [CI], 0.10 to 1.38) and number of episodes of suicidal acts (1.88 compared with 3.03; MD 1.26; 95% CI, -0.06 to 2.58).[40, 41]

Linehan and colleagues (2006) investigated the effectiveness of a DBT intervention versus community treatment by experts in a sample of 111 adult women.[38] However, as there were no suicide deaths in this trial, there is insufficient evidence to draw conclusions about the relative effectiveness of suicide death prevention. The study provides low strength evidence of a significantly lower suicide attempt rate for DBT (23.1% compared with 46%; Hazard ratio [HR] 2.66, $p = .005$).

Another study of DBT by McMain and colleagues (2009) compared the treatment to general psychiatric management.[42] Similar to the evidence from the Linehan et al. (2006) study, this trial provides insufficient evidence to draw conclusions about differential effects on risk of suicide death due to a lack of observed events. However, this study provides low strength evidence for a non-significant treatment effect on mean number of suicide attempts and self-harm at 12 months (4.29 compared with 12.87).

Psychotherapy Interventions for People with Recent Suicide Attempts, Recent Self-Harm Incidents, or Imminent Risk

Psychotherapy results reported in the Mann et al. systematic review included insufficient to low strength evidence supporting the suicidal self-directed violence preventive effects of cognitive therapies, interpersonal psychotherapy, and problem-solving therapy. Notably, these results were presented in the Mann et al. report as coming from very few studies with small sample sizes, methodological flaws, and short-term follow-up assessment periods, suggesting that all findings are of insufficient to low strength and should be interpreted with caution.

We included seven RCTs of psychotherapy interventions for people with recent suicide attempts, recent self-harm incidents, or imminent risk.[36, 43-45, 47, 48, 50] Only three of the trials reported an assessment of suicide deaths, but all provided only insufficient to low strength evidence because of lack of statistical power and methodological flaws.[43-45]

A large (N = 1094) RCT conducted by Hatcher and colleagues (2011) in New Zealand provided moderate strength of evidence of a non-significant effect of problem-solving treatment plus treatment as usual versus treatment as usual on the outcomes of re-presentation to the hospital for self-harm (14.2% vs 17.1%; Relative risk [RR] 0.17; 95% CI, -0.24 to 0.44) and self-reported self-harm (27.4% vs 32.7%; RR 0.16; 95% CI, -0.13 to 0.38).[36] However, the authors also report examination of an a priori hypothesis to see whether there were different treatment effects for patients whose index hospitalization was the first time they were hospitalized for self-harm behavior versus patients who were repeatedly hospitalized for self-harm behavior prior to the intervention. They report that the treatment showed no significant effect in patients who were hospitalized for the first time; however, there were significantly fewer re-presentations to the hospital for self-harm behaviors for both consenting and all (consenting and non-consenting, i.e., ITT analysis) patients when only patients who had repeated hospitalizations for self-harm prior to the intervention were considered. There were also significantly fewer participants who self-reported engaging in self-harm behaviors from the group of consenting patients when only patients who had repeated hospitalizations for self-harm prior to the intervention were considered, though this self-report data was not able to be obtained from non-consenting patients for the ITT analysis. The authors report that analyses adjusting for treatment location and therapist nesting had no effect on the results. Finally, a similar pattern of statistically significant results for patient groups was reported for time to re-presentation to the hospital for self-harm behaviors, with patients hospitalized for repeat self-harm in the treatment group showing a significant improvement in time to re-presentation when compared to patients in the control condition; these results were significant for both consenting patients as well as the combined group of consenting and non-consenting patients (i.e., the ITT analysis).

We also included RCTs that compared CAMS versus E-CAU in a population of adults with a recent suicide attempt or imminent risk,[47] a skills-based intervention versus a supportive therapy control condition,[48] CBT compared to problem solving therapy compared to treatment as usual,[50] and intensive case management with a therapy component,[45] but all trials provided insufficient evidence to draw conclusions about self-directed violence prevention due to an unacceptably high risk of bias.

A study of Attachment-Based Family Therapy versus Enhanced Usual Care resulted in fewer low lethality suicide attempts in the treatment condition (11% in the treatment and 22% in the control group), though a low strength evidence rating limits the ability to draw a firm conclusion about the results.[46]

Notably, a study of group therapy for adolescents between 12 and 16 years of age resulted in an 88 percent incidence of repeated self-harm after 12 months compared to a 71 percent incidence of self-harm ($p = .07$) in the routine care condition, indicating the possibility of iatrogenic effects in the group treatment condition. This study provided low strength evidence, however, and, therefore, conclusions about the possibility of iatrogenic effects are tentative.[49] Another, more recent study of group therapy conducted by Green and colleagues provides low strength evidence,[44] though in spite of a relatively large sample size (N = 366), this study reported no suicide deaths among all participants, and only one incident of self-harm with severe injury in the treatment group compared to two instances in the control group.

Psychotherapy Interventions for People with a Psychotic Spectrum Disorder

We included one RCT that compared CBT with supportive counseling in 278 participants.[51]
However, despite the relatively large sample size, this trial had an unacceptably high risk of bias
and provided insufficient evidence to draw conclusions about the relative effectiveness of the two
treatments in self-directed violence prevention.

Psychotherapy Interventions for People with Depression or Dysthymia

An RCT of the IMPACT intervention included a comprehensive depression case management
and treatment component compared to usual care in a population of adults age 60 and older.[52]
In spite of the large sample size of this trial (N=1801) with unclear risk of bias, it provides
insufficient evidence to draw conclusions about differential effects on risk of suicide death due to
a lack of observed events.

KEY QUESTION #3. What is the effectiveness of referral and follow-up services (e.g., strategies designed to provide referrals, improve referral follow-through and attendance, etc.) for reducing rates of suicidal self-directed violence in military and/or Veteran populations?

We did not find any new RCTs on self-directed violence referral and follow-up services in
military and/or VA health care settings.

KEY QUESTION #4. What lessons can be learned from research on self-directed violence referral and follow-up services conducted outside of VA or military settings that can be applied to Veteran and/or military populations?

Summary of Findings

The three previously published reports on this topic all report overall insufficient to low strength
of evidence for the effectiveness of any referral and follow-up services in prevention of self-
directed violence.[9-11] Specific findings from the three reports include positive results from studies
on case management/care coordination and 24-hour contact with a mental health professional.
Mixed reports of findings came from studies on emergency contact cards and postal contact. Null
findings were reported from studies investigating intensive psychosocial follow-up, telephone
follow-up, and video education plus family therapy. Notably, these results were presented in the
previous reports as coming from very few studies with small sample sizes, many methodological
flaws, and short-term follow-up assessment periods, suggesting that all findings are of
insufficient to low strength and should be interpreted with caution.

Of the primary studies included in this review, three studies of postcard interventions to decrease
repeated self-harm showed mixed results.[53-55] Two studies of Youth-Nominated Support Team
(YST) interventions combined with usual care did not significantly reduce risk of suicide
attempts or death in suicidal adolescents.[56, 57] One study of assertive community treatment
compared with community mental health care in difficult-to-engage adults with serious mental

illness showed no reduction in suicide deaths or deliberate self-harm incidents.[58] Finally, one trial of a depression care management program resulted in no significant changes in the suicide mortality rate of older adults in primary care settings.[59] However, all these studies were given low strength of evidence ratings and thus limit conclusions about the effectiveness of these interventions.

Studies of Efficacy

Systematic Reviews

We identified nine new systematic reviews relevant to referral and follow-up services published in 10 articles subsequent to Mann 2005.[14, 90, 96, 103, 106, 109, 112, 115, 118, 119] Of these, six were rated high quality according to the Oxman and Guyatt validation index[15] and are included in the summary below.[14, 106, 109, 112, 115, 118] Three were rated lower quality and are not discussed further in this report.

Of the six high quality systematic reviews, three included only primary studies that were outside the scope of this review: primary studies with a broader range of studies designs (i.e., observational studies); publication dates (i.e., before 2005); and from a broader range of countries than our focus on the US, United Kingdom, Canada, New Zealand, and Australia. The other three high quality systematic reviews included a total of three eligible RCTs.[54, 55, 58] Therefore, we were only able to use existing new reviews as an additional source of identifying new primary RCTs. These three RCTs are included as primary studies in our review.

Appendices T and U present quality assessment of the systematic reviews and data abstraction of the primary studies obtained from the systematic reviews.

Three previously published reports on this topic with similar key questions to the current report all report findings of referral and follow-up services with different combinations of studies into categories, making comparisons across reports difficult.[9-11] Results are reported in Appendix V, and all three reports note the overall insufficient to low strength of evidence for the effectiveness of any referral and follow-up services in prevention of self-directed violence. Specific findings from the three reports include positive results from studies on case management/care coordination and 24-hour contact with a mental health professional. Mixed reports of findings came from studies on emergency contact cards and postal contact. Null findings were reported from studies investigating intensive psychosocial follow-up, telephone follow-up, and video education plus family therapy. Notably, these results were presented in the three systematic reviews as coming from very few studies with small sample sizes, methodological flaws, and short-term follow-up assessment periods, suggesting that all findings are of insufficient to low strength and should be interpreted with caution. The findings from the Mann et al. report, which was conducted with a similar search strategy to this report with non-overlapping search dates, are combined with the results from our search and presented in the following results section and associated tables.

Randomized Controlled Trials (RCTs)

Appendices X through Z present data abstraction, risk of bias assessment, and strength of evidence grading of the primary studies included in this review.

We also report a summary of sample sizes, outcome definitions, and results from all RCTs included in this review along with a description of the purpose of the study in order to examine possible relationships among study intent and design, and outcome. Of particular interest was whether studies which were designed to treat suicidal self-directed violence might be better powered to detect effects of such a low base rate outcome when compared to studies designed to treat another related but more common outcome such as depression. These results are presented in Appendix W for studies investigating referral and follow-up services. Notably, there does not appear to be a strong relationship between sample size (and, by extension, statistical power) and whether or not the studies were reportedly designed to treat suicidal self-directed violence versus other outcomes.

Postcard Interventions

The Mann review included one RCT of 843 persons which found a significantly lower suicide rate for at least two years in those who were contacted by letter at least four times a year compared to those who received no further contact after discharge following hospitalization due to a depressive or suicidal state.[10] This trial provides insufficient to low strength evidence for the effectiveness of postcard interventions in preventing suicidal self-directed violence.

However, findings from two RCTs (in three publications) with unclear risk of bias provided low strength evidence of mixed results regarding effects of postcard interventions on repeat self-harm.[53-55] In 772 adults discharged from a Newcastle, Australia hospital after deliberate self-poisoning, compared to standard treatment alone, eight postcards sent over 12 months significantly reduced the cumulative number of repeat episodes of deliberate self-poisoning both at 12 months (Incident Risk Ratio [IRR] 0.55; 95% CI, 0.35 to 0.87) and at 24 months (IRR 0.49; 95% CI, 0.33 to 0.73), but did not reduce the proportion of patients with repeat deliberate self-poisoning at either time point.[54, 55] However, at both 12 months and 24 months, subgroup analyses found that the significant reduction in cumulative number of repeat episodes of deliberate self-poisoning with the postcard intervention was observed only in women and not in men.

In a later trial of 327 individuals aged 16 and older who were discharged from Christchurch Hospital in New Zealand following self-harm of attempted suicide, compared to treatment as usual and after adjustment for prior self-harm, six postcards mailed over 12 months did not significantly reduce the total number of self-harm re-presentations (IRR 1.07; 95% CI, 0.80 to 1.43) or total proportion of patients who re-presented for self-harm (OR 0.97; 95% CI, 0.58 to 1.62).[53]

Youth-Nominated Support Team (YST)

The Mann review did not include any RCTs of YST interventions.[10] However, we found two RCTs with unclear risk of bias that provided low-strength evidence that, compared to treatment as usual only, adding YST did not significantly reduce suicide deaths or attempts in suicidal, psychiatrically hospitalized adolescents in the US.[56, 57]

In general, the YST intervention supplements usual care by providing youth-nominated support persons who maintain regular contact with the patients following hospitalization. In the first trial, YST-I, adolescents had the option of including one peer in the support team and the regular contact was maintained for six months, but there was a trend toward a higher proportion of patients with one or more suicide attempts in the YST group (17.3%) compared to the treatment as usual only group (11.6%, P=0.26).[57] In the second trial, YST-II, the support team was limited to adults only and contact was only maintained for three months, which led to a slightly lower number of patients with at least one suicide attempt in the YST group (13% compared with 15%, P=0.51).[56]

Assertive Community Treatment

The Mann review did not include any RCTs of assertive community treatment.[10] However, we found one RCT with unclear risk of bias that provided low-strength evidence that, compared to care from a community mental health team, assertive community treatment did not significantly reduce suicide deaths (0.8% compared with 2.5%; P not reported) or deliberate self-harm incidents (8% compared with 11%, P=0.40) over 18 months among 251 adults with serious mental illness and identified as having difficulty engaging with standard community care.[58] This trial was conducted in London, and the assertive community treatment approach involved smaller case loads than carried by the community mental health teams and all team members worked with all clients, met at up to a daily frequency for discussion, used assertive contact with clients, followed a "no drop-out" policy, and offered extended hours of availability, and "in vivo" locations for appointments.

Case Management/Care Coordination

The Mann review[10] reported fewer suicide attempts compared to control participants from one study investigating the use of a suicide intervention counselor providing care coordination/case management services; however, this information was not from an RCT and is, therefore, not included in the findings for this current report.

However, we identified a more recent secondary analysis of suicide deaths[59] from the trial of older primary care patients originally included in the Mann review.[120] The Prevention of Suicide in Primary Care Elderly: Collaborative Trial (PROSPECT) had unclear risk of bias and compared the effect of algorithm-based depression care management to usual care practices in 599 older primary care patients with major depression (age ≥ 60 years). PROSPECT provided low-strength evidence that algorithm-based depression care management did not significantly change the suicide mortality rate per 1,000 person-years overall (0.7 [95% CI, 0.0 to 4.2] compared with 0.0 [95% CI, 0.0 to 3.3]), or in subgroups with either major depressive disorder (N=396: 0.0 [95% CI, 0.0 to 4.1] compared with 0.0 [95% CI, 0.0 to 5.1]), or clinically significant minor depression (N=203: 2.2 [95% CI, 0.1 to 2.5] compared with 0.0 [95% CI, 0.0 to 9.7]).

Emergency Contact Card Interventions

The Mann review included one RCT of an emergency contact card intervention, and reported a reduced rate of suicide attempts.[10] This trial provides insufficient to lowstrength evidence for the effectiveness of emergency contact interventions in preventing suicidal self-directed violence.

SUMMARY AND DISCUSSION

Suicide is an extraordinarily complex phenomenon, associated with a range of demographic, biological, psycho-social, and clinical risk factors. Despite the number of risk factors, any given person's individual risk for suicide or suicide attempt is low.[78] The complex nature of factors contributing to suicide and the relatively low population rate make interventions challenging. The complexity of suicide is reflected in the diversity of research aimed at understanding and preventing suicidal behaviors. For this review, we evaluated the evidence from RCTs of interventions aimed at reducing suicide and suicide attempts. We found articles reporting on a broad range of interventions from pharmacotherapy to psychotherapy and case management in patient populations of all ages. However, we found very few trials specifically evaluating interventions in Veteran and military populations.

Our initial searches yielded nearly 16,500 titles published on suicide treatments and risk factors since 2005. From these we identified 45 RCTs and 40 systematic reviews that provided evidence for specific treatment interventions, or referral and follow-up strategies to reduce rates of suicidal self-directed violence. Interventions included antidepressants, antipsychotics, mood stabilizers, omega-3 fatty acid supplements, CBT, and DBT, among others. Follow-up and referral strategies included postcard interventions, YSTs, and assertive community treatment. Overall, these intervention trials had methodological limitations that resulted in their providing only low strength and insufficient evidence to properly draw conclusions on the effectiveness of the various treatment interventions and follow-up/referral strategies. No interventions stood out as clearly more effective than others. This review did not evaluate any outcomes other than suicidal self-directed violence and, therefore, no additional data on potential harms and side effects was investigated.

While the gold standard for testing interventions is an RCT, the majority of the literature documenting efforts to reduce suicidal behaviors is observational in nature, and lacking in comparison or control conditions. Although information from such studies can be extremely valuable, it can also be misleading due to the potential for participant, provider, or researcher expectations about the effectiveness of the treatment under investigation to inflate positive results. As the goal of this report was to summarize the best evidence available, we focused on RCTs to minimize the risk of inflated positive results. Further, because of the noted inadequacies of proxy outcomes such as suicidal ideation for studying suicidal behavior,[121] we limited our included studies to those that reported self-directed violence behaviors, specifically suicide and suicide attempts, as well as self-directed violence with undetermined intent. Though extensive observational research has been conducted on the natural course of suicide in a variety of populations including Veterans and members of the military, few RCTs have been conducted investigating the effectiveness of interventions or referral and follow-up services on reducing suicide or suicide attempts. Though a thorough review of unpublished and ongoing research is outside the scope of this report, some reviewers suggested that there is such research currently being conducted by VA investigators. The paucity of RCT research is likely due to the difficulty of studying an outcome with such low base rates, even in the highest risk populations.

As noted, we found 38 RCTs that satisfied our inclusion criteria and reported outcome data on suicides or suicide attempts. In spite of this relatively large number of trials, the data obtained provided only low strength or insufficient evidence to draw conclusions about the effectiveness of the interventions and referral/follow-up services being studied. This is primarily because interventions provided, populations studied, and comparison conditions examined in the 45 were so heterogeneous. This heterogeneity precluded meaningful comparisons across trials and quantitative combination of results from multiple trials. Therefore, each trial essentially stands alone for providing evidence related to the specific intervention being investigated. For example, though multiple studies compared psychotherapeutic interventions broadly categorized as either DBT or CBT, some studied a solely female population and all used different comparison conditions, making the combination of findings impossible.

Though large, high quality trials have the potential to stand alone as strong evidence, this was not the case with the 38 trials included in this systematic review. One limitation was inadequate blinding. Although some RCTs are more straightforward and can be easily conducted with adequate blinding techniques (e.g., pharmacological studies), many interventions and referral/follow-up services appropriate for suicide prevention are difficult if not impossible to blind in a study. Ideally, patients would be unaware of their treatment/control group status, and providers would be unaware of treatment/control group status. Also, in the case of psychotherapeutic interventions, providers' belief and expertise in providing a particular type of intervention is paramount to its effectiveness – so blinding is even more essential than it is with a pharmacologic study. Despite this challenge, it is possible to compare psychotherapeutic interventions in adequately blinded studies. An adequately blinded study would involve therapists who are experts in each of the reputable and presumably effective treatments being compared. The evaluation of effectiveness would be conducted by someone who was unaware of the intervention. For example, despite other sources of bias, the Linehan (2006) study investigating DBT provides a good example of an intervention comparison in which both patients and providers could reasonably assume that the treatments being delivered are effective.[38] Thus, the risk of bias due to inadequate provider confidence in the therapy (a problem when the provider knows that he/she is delivering the placebo intervention) was minimized. These trials still require independent assessment of the outcome, though from the patient-provider standpoint, this is an example of a reasonably well-blinded study. Most RCTs of interventions and referral/ follow-up services found in this report, however, did not utilize adequate blinding procedures or comparison conditions. This inadequacy undermines the validity of the study results since patients and/or providers were likely aware of treatment assignment.

In addition to deficiencies in study design quality, a major reason that many of the trials in this report were unable to provide higher strength evidence for their findings was because they were insufficiently powered to detect an effect of the intervention. This is not uncommon when the outcome being studied has a low base rate. In many of the studies reviewed here, sample sizes were very small (in the 40s) and it is not surprising that these trials did not show any difference in outcomes between the groups. Although some trials were significantly larger, even the largest trials included in this review with sample sizes of over 1,000 participants resulted in an under-powered study design.

The issue of low base rate impacting sample size and overall strength of evidence also extends to the generalizability of the trials included in this report. For example, most of the trials included in this report examined populations with existing mental health diagnoses. This was necessary from a design standpoint in order to have a population with a reasonable likelihood of demonstrating a difference in the outcome between the interventions being studied. Though members of the military and Veterans may have mental health diagnoses, the Veteran and military population in general is not solely comprised of people with mental health diagnoses and, therefore, these results do not necessarily represent the entire Veteran and military population. Other studies applied very stringent exclusion criteria in order to have a more homogeneous participant pool, or for safety reasons due to the outcome of interest. This practice, though necessary at times, can limit generalizability and also make detection of an effect even more difficult due to the exclusion of patients with higher rates of suicidal self-directed violence.

There are many different paths to suicide, and there are many unique risk and protective factors that are difficult to study in non-Veteran/military populations. For example, we found no RCTs investigating the effectiveness of interventions to reduce self-directed violence in people diagnosed with Posttraumatic Stress Disorder or Traumatic Brain Injury, two disorders very common among Veterans and members of the military. Life stressors may be very different for this population of interest because of the duties they perform in the line of duty, the time they are potentially required to spend away from family and other support systems, and the potentially protective factors related to being a part of an organization like the military.

LIMITATIONS

The lack of high quality trials is not a limitation of this review, per se, but rather a reflection of the available literature. However, in spite of finding few trials for our questions related to Veteran and military populations, we did not examine observational and uncontrolled studies. We felt that the best available evidence would come from trials conducted in non-Veteran/military populations rather than from observational studies conducted with our population of interest due to the inherent limitations in ability to ascribe causality to findings from non-experimental studies and studies lacking adequate control conditions. We also chose to limit the outcomes considered in this review to suicidal self-directed violence, which does not include suicidal ideation. This scoping decision could result in the exclusion of some studies related to suicidal self-directed violence if they did not collect and report data on that outcome. This review did not evaluate any outcomes other than suicidal self-directed violence, and, therefore, no additional data on potential harms and side effects were investigated. Potential harms and side effects should always be considered when evaluating the strength of evidence and considering adoption of an intervention or referral/follow-up service. Finally, it is likely that our search strategy, though based on previous systematic reviews on this topic, could have been more comprehensive and, therefore, some studies could have been left out of this review. For example, some reviewers noted that studies on other types of violent death (e.g., homicide) may have been left out of this search, even though the topics could be highly related.

RECOMMENDATIONS FOR FUTURE RESEARCH

Due to the low base rate of the primary outcome of interest in suicide, as well as in the complexity of many of the commonly implemented interventions for suicide prevention, high quality RCTs are difficult to implement. In spite of this difficulty, however, there remains a need to further test existing and new treatment methods that could be effective in preventing suicide.

A few high quality RCTs of promising interventions could change the strength of evidence for those interventions. Additionally, large-scale studies are needed to more effectively address unanswered questions about suicide because of its low base rates. Many studies included in this report cited a lack of research funding and support for the type of large-scale clinical trials needed to investigate an outcome with such low base-rates. Though the expense might be great, well-designed, very large-scale, multi-site trials with the capability to collect data on a sufficiently large population are needed to more adequately answer questions about the effectiveness of interventions designed to decrease suicide rates. Though small-scale trials may provide important information about intervention feasibility, resources might be best spent on very large-scale investigations of the most promising interventions in order to conduct adequately powered studies that have the ability to detect an intervention effect.

Other reviews have examined common elements of the most promising suicide prevention interventions, and such non-systematic reviewing of literature could be used to help guide future research in this area.[122] This field still needs investigation of interventions and referral/follow-up services that are specifically targeted to be applicable to members of the military and Veteran populations. Additionally, when considering future research as well as intervention adoption, researchers and clinicians should consider intervention costs and potential harms; these two issues were outside the scope of this review, though the articles cited reported little information on these topics, suggesting that these are areas in need of further investigation.

Given the overall limited evidence from the interventions described in this report, it is important to identify the relatively most promising interventions to help guide future research. One of the most promising interventions, Problem Solving Therapy, was reported in the Hatcher et al. study.[36] This one study, conducted outside the US with a non-military/Veteran population, provides only moderate strength evidence for self-directed violence preventive effects in a specific sub-population of patients admitted to the hospital with repeated self-harm. Additionally, the findings from this current report combined with the findings from an earlier systematic review[10] suggest that DBT has low strength evidence for effectiveness in self-directed violence prevention in populations with Borderline Personality Disorder. These interventions might be well-suited to future trials in VA and military settings to add to the overall evidence base, and to determine effectiveness in Veteran and military populations.

CONCLUSIONS

Examining RCTs of interventions is the gold standard for determining relative efficacy. Though there are some RCTs of suicide prevention interventions, these trials are largely plagued by study design flaws and insufficient power. This is likely due to: a) the complexity of conducting high quality trials of interventions that involve psychotherapy, and b) the very low base rates of suicide and suicide attempts even in the highest risk groups. In our systematic review of the evidence related to suicide prevention interventions, we found these two issues to be paramount to the lack of strong evidence for any interventions in preventing suicide and suicide attempts.

We were most interested in RCTs related to Veteran and military populations as stated in Key Questions #1 and #3; however, we found no such trials meeting our inclusion criteria published since 2005. We, therefore, examined trials in non-Veteran/military populations in the hopes of generalizing findings to our populations of interest. The included studies covered a broad range of interventions implemented with various populations in terms of gender, age, and diagnosis. Even the broader inclusion criteria of Key Questions #2 and #4 did not provide clear answers as to which interventions or referrals and follow-up services are most effective in the prevention of suicidal or undetermined self-directed violence. Therefore, it is likely the best available evidence for interventions to prevent suicide is to use a combination of the most theoretically sound and well researched interventions available. For example, if a Veteran or member of the military is identified as being at risk for suicide, making sure that this person has adequate case management to assist with intervention attendance as well as family or other social support outside of the medical setting are both likely to be good clinical practice. Additionally, assuring that the individual has access to relatively immediate care such as inpatient hospitalization, outpatient therapy, and pharmacotherapy is also warranted depending on the individual's level of risk. Finally, providers should take into consideration which interventions are most likely to benefit the individual based on diagnosis or other relevant clinical factors (e.g., use of mood stabilizers if a patient meets criteria for Bipolar Disorder, or referral to an emotion regulation-focused psychotherapy intervention such as DBT if the patient meets criteria for Borderline Personality Disorder). Overall, the intervention and referral/follow-up service studies that were included in this report were quite complex and appeared very comprehensive in nature; such a comprehensive and multifaceted approach to suicide prevention care for Veterans and members of the military appears well warranted.

REFERENCES

1.   Kochanek KD, Xu J, Murphy SL, Miniño AM, Kung H-C. Deaths: preliminary data for 2009. *Natl Vital Stat Rep.* 2011;59(4):1-51.

2.   Centers for Disease Control and Prevention, National Center for Injury Prevention and Control. National Violent Death Reporting System: Monitoring and Tracking the Causes of Violent Deaths - 2008. 2008; http://www.cdph.ca.gov/programs/Documents/nvdrs_aag_2008-a.pdf. Accessed February 29, 2012.

3.   McCarthy JF, Valenstein M, Kim HM, Ilgen M, Zivin K, Blow FC. Suicide mortality among patients receiving care in the veterans health administration health system. *American journal of epidemiology.* 2009 Apr 15;169(8):1033-8.

4.   Department of Veterans Affairs. Screening and evaluation of possible traumatic brain injury in operation enduring freedom (OEF) and operation Iraqi freedom (OIF) veterans. *VHA Directive 2007-013.* 2007.

5.   Department of Veterans Affairs. Report of the Blue Ribbon Work Group on Suicide Prevention in the Veteran Population. 2008; Available at http://www.mentalhealth.va.gov/suicide_prevention/Blue_Ribbon_Report-FINAL_June-30-08.pdf. Accessed January 3, 2012.

6.   US Public Health Service. *The Surgeon General's Call to Action to Prevent Suicide.* Washington, D.C.1999.

7.   World Health Organization. SUPRE Prevention of suicidal behaviors: a task for all. 2007; Available at http://www.who.int/mental_health/prevention/suicide/information/en/index.html. Accessed January 3, 2012.

8.   Nock MK, Borges G, Bromet EJ, Cha CB, Kessler RC, Lee S. Suicide and suicidal behavior. *Epidemiol Rev.* 2008;30:133-54.

9.   Gaynes BN, West SL, Ford CA, et al. Screening for Suicide Risk in Adults: A Summary of the Evidence for the U.S. Preventive Services Task Force. *Annals of Internal Medicine May.* 2004;140(10):822-35.

10. Mann JJ, Apter A, Bertolote J, et al. Suicide prevention strategies: a systematic review. *JAMA.* 2005 Oct 26;294(16):2064-74.

11. National Institute for Health and Clinical Excellence. Self-harm: longer-term management in adults, children and young people [Draft for Consultation]. *National Collaborating Centre for Mental Health,.* 2011.

12. Centers for Disease Control and Prevention, Crosby AE, Han B, et al. Suicidal thoughts and behaviors among adults aged ≥18 years --- United States, 2008-2009. *MMWR Surveill Summ.* 2011 Oct 21;60(13):1-22.

13. Brenner LA, Breshears RE, Betthauser LM, et al. Implementation of a Suicide Nomenclature within Two VA Healthcare Settings. *J Clin Psychol Med Settings.* 2011 Jun;18(2):116-28.

14. Shekelle P, Bagley S, Munjas B. Strategies for Suicide Prevention in Veterans. *Evidence-based Synthesis Program.* 2009 Jan.

15. Oxman AD, Guyatt GH. Validation of an index of the quality of review articles. *Journal of Clinical Epidemiology.* 1991;44(11):1271-8.

16. Higgins J, Green S. *Cochrane Handbook for Systematic Reviews of Interventions Version 5.1.0.* [updated March 2011]. Available from www.cochrane-handbook.org; 2011.

17. Owens DK, Lohr KN, Atkins D, et al. AHRQ series paper 5: grading the strength of a body of evidence when comparing medical interventions--agency for healthcare research and quality and the effective health-care program. *J Clin Epidemiol.* 2010 May;63(5):513-23.

18. Emslie GJ, Wagner KD, Kutcher S, et al. Paroxetine treatment in children and adolescents with major depressive disorder: a randomized, multicenter, double-blind, placebo-controlled trial. *Journal of the American Academy of Child & Adolescent Psychiatry.* 2006;45(6):709-19.

19. Emslie G, Kratochvil C, Vitiello B, et al. Treatment for Adolescents with Depression Study (TADS): safety results. *J Am Acad Child Adolesc Psychiatry.* 2006 Dec;45(12):1440-55.

20. Emslie GJ, Ventura D, Korotzer A, Tourkodimitris S. Escitalopram in the treatment of adolescent depression: A randomized placebo-controlled multisite trial. *Journal of the American Academy of Child & Adolescent Psychiatry.* 2009 Jul;48(7):721-9.

21. March JS, Silva S, Petrycki S, et al. The Treatment for Adolescents With Depression Study (TADS): long-term effectiveness and safety outcomes. *Arch Gen Psychiatry.* 2007 Oct;64(10):1132-43.

22. Wagner KD, Jonas J, Findling RL, Ventura D, Saikali K. A double-blind, randomized, placebo-controlled trial of escitalopram in the treatment of pediatric depression. *J Am Acad Child Adolesc Psychiatry.* 2006 Mar;45(3):280-8.

23. DeRubeis RJ, Hollon SD, Amsterdam JD, et al. Cognitive therapy vs medications in the treatment of moderate to severe depression. *Archives of General Psychiatry.* 2005;62(4):409-16.

24. Grunebaum MF, Ellis SP, Duan N, Burke AK, Oquendo MA, John Mann J. Pilot Randomized Clinical Trial of an SSRI vs Bupropion: Effects on Suicidal Behavior, Ideation, and Mood in Major Depression. *Neuropsychopharmacology.* 2011 Oct 12.

25. Zisook S, Lesser IM, Lebowitz B, et al. Effect of antidepressant medication treatment on suicidal ideation and behavior in a randomized trial: an exploratory report from the Combining Medications to Enhance Depression Outcomes Study. *J Clin Psychiatry.* 2011 Oct;72(10):1322-32.

26. Brent DA, Emslie GJ, Clarke GN, et al. Predictors of spontaneous and systematically assessed suicidal adverse events in the treatment of SSRI-resistant depression in adolescents (TORDIA) study. *Am J Psychiatry.* 2009 Apr;166(4):418-26.

27. Goodyer IM, Dubicka B, Wilkinson P, et al. A randomised controlled trial of cognitive behaviour therapy in adolescents with major depression treated by selective serotonin reuptake inhibitors. The ADAPT trial. *Health Technol Assess.* 2008 May;12(14):iii-iv, ix-60.

28. Calabrese J, Keck P, Macfadden W, et al. A randomized, double-blind, placebo-controlled trial of quetiapine in the treatment of Bipolar I or II depression. *Am J Psychiatry.* 2005;162:1351-60.

29. Berman RM, Marcus RN, Swanink R, et al. The efficacy and safety of aripiprazole as adjunctive therapy in major depressive disorder: a multicenter, randomized, double-blind, placebo-controlled study. *Journal of Clinical Psychiatry.* 2007;68(6):843-53.

30. Marcus RN, McQuade RD, Carson WH, et al. The efficacy and safety of aripiprazole as adjunctive therapy in major depressive disorder: a second multicenter, randomized, double-blind, placebo-controlled study. *Journal of Clinical Psychopharmacology.* 2008;28(2):156-65.

31. Weisler RH, Khan A, Trivedi MH, et al. Analysis of suicidality in pooled data from 2 double-blind, placebo-controlled aripiprazole adjunctive therapy trials in major depressive disorder. *J Clin Psychiatry.* 2011 Apr;72(4):548-55.

32. Oquendo M, Galfalvy H, Currier D, et al. Treatment of suicide attempters with bipolar disorder: a randomized clinical trial comparing lithium and valproate in the prevention of suicidal behavior. *Am J Psychiatry.* 2011;168(10):1050-6.

33. Khan A, Khan SR, Hobus J, et al. Differential pattern of response in mood symptoms and suicide risk measures in severely ill depressed patients assigned to citalopram with placebo or citalopram combined with lithium: Role of lithium levels. *J Psychiatr Res.* 2011 Nov;45(11):1489-96.

34. Lauterbach E, Felber W, Muller-Oerlinghausen B, et al. Adjunctive lithium treatment in the prevention of suicidal behaviour in depressive disorders: a randomised, placebo-controlled, 1-year trial. *Acta Psychiatr Scand.* 2008 Dec;118(6):469-79.

35. Hallahan B, Hibbeln JR, Davis JM, Garland MR. Omega-3 fatty acid supplementation in patients with recurrent self-harm. Single-centre double-blind randomised controlled trial. *NA.* 2007;190:118-22.

36. Hatcher S, Sharon C, Parag V, Collins N. Problem-solving therapy for people who present to hospital with self-harm: Zelen randomised controlled trial. *Br J Psychiatry.* 2011 Oct;199:310-6.

37. Bateman A, Fonagy P. Randomized controlled trial of outpatient mentalization-based treatment versus structured clinical management for borderline personality disorder. *Am J Psychiatry.* 2009 Dec;166(12):1355-64.

38. Linehan MM, Comtois KA, Murray AM, et al. Two-year randomized controlled trial and follow-up of dialectical behavior therapy vs therapy by experts for suicidal behaviors and borderline personality disorder. *Arch Gen Psychiatry.* 2006 Jul;63(7):757-66.

39. Blum N, St John D, Pfohl B, et al. Systems Training for Emotional Predictability and Problem Solving (STEPPS) for outpatients with borderline personality disorder: a randomized controlled trial and 1-year follow-up [erratum appears in Am J Psychiatry 165(6): 777]. *Am J Psychiatry.* 2008 Apr;165(4):468-78.

40. Davidson K, Norrie J, Tyrer P, et al. The effectiveness of cognitive behavior therapy for borderline personality disorder: results from the borderline personality disorder study of cognitive therapy (BOSCOT) trial. *J Pers Disord.* 2006 Oct;20(5):450-65.

41. Davidson KM, Tyrer P, Norrie J, Palmer SJ, Tyrer H. Cognitive therapy v. usual treatment for borderline personality disorder: prospective 6-year follow-up. *Br J Psychiatry.* 2010 Dec;197:456-62.

42. McMain SF, Links PS, Gnam WH, et al. A randomized trial of dialectical behavior therapy versus general psychiatric management for borderline personality disorder. *Am J Psychiatry.* 2009 Dec;166(12):1365-74.

43. Winter D, Sireling L, Riley T, Metcalfe C, Quaite A, Bhandari S. A controlled trial of personal construct psychotherapy for deliberate self-harm. *Psychology and Psychotherapy: Theory, Research and Practice.* 2007 Mar;80(1):23-37.

44. Green JM, Wood AJ, Kerfoot MJ, et al. Group therapeutic treatment for adolescents with repeated self harm (assist) – a randomised controlled trial with economic evaluation. *BMJ.* 2011;342:682-.

45. De Leo D, Heller T. Intensive case management in suicide attempters following discharge from inpatient psychiatric care. *Australian Journal of Primary Health.* 2007;13(3):49-58.

46. Diamond GS, Wintersteen MB, Brown GK, et al. Attachment-based family therapy for adolescents with suicidal ideation: A randomized controlled trial. [References]. *Journal of the American Academy of Child & Adolescent Psychiatry.* 2010;49(2):122-31.

47. Comtois KA, Jobes DA, S SOC, et al. Collaborative assessment and management of suicidality (CAMS): feasibility trial for next-day appointment services. *Depress Anxiety.* 2011 Sep 21.

48. Donaldson D, Spirito A, Esposito-Smythers C. Treatment for Adolescents Following a Suicide Attempt: Results of a Pilot Trial. *Journal of the American Academy of Child & Adolescent Psychiatry.* 2005 Feb;44(2):113-20.

49. Hazell PL, Martin G, McGill K, et al. Group therapy for repeated deliberate self-harm in adolescents: failure of replication of a randomized trial. *Journal of the American Academy of Child & Adolescent Psychiatry.* 2009 Jun;48(6):662-70.

50. Stewart CD, Quinn A, Plever S, Emmerson B. Comparing cognitive behavior therapy, problem solving therapy, and treatment as usual in a high risk population. *Suicide Life Threat Behav.* 2009 Oct;39(5):538-47.

51. Tarrier N, Haddock G, Lewis S, Drake R, Gregg L, So CTG. Suicide behaviour over 18 months in recent onset schizophrenic patients: the effects of CBT. *Schizophr Res.* 2006 Mar;83(1):15-27.

52. Unutzer J, Tang L, Oishi S, et al. Reducing suicidal ideation in depressed older primary care patients. *J Am Geriatr Soc.* 2006 Oct;54(10):1550-6.

53. Beautrais AL, Gibb SJ, Faulkner A, Fergusson DM, Mulder RT. Postcard intervention for repeat self-harm: randomised controlled trial. *NA.* 2010 Jul;197(1):55-60.

54. Carter GL, Clover K, Whyte IM, Dawson AH, D'Este C. Postcards from the EDge project: Randomised controlled trial of an intervention using postcards to reduce repetition of hospital treated deliberate self poisoning. *BMJ.* 2005 Oct;331(7520):805.

55. Carter GL, Clover K, Whyte IM, Dawson AH, D'Este C. Postcards from the EDge: 24-month outcomes of a randomised controlled trial for hospital-treated self-poisoning. *British Journal of Psychiatry.* 2007;191:548-53.

56. King CA, Klaus N, Kramer A, Venkataraman S, Quinlan P, Gillespie B. The Youth-Nominated Support Team-Version II for suicidal adolescents: A randomized controlled intervention trial. *J Consult Clin Psychol.* 2009 Oct;77(5):880-93.

57. King CA, Kramer A, Preuss L, Kerr DC, Weisse L, Venkataraman S. Youth-Nominated Support Team for Suicidal Adolescents (Version 1): a randomized controlled trial. *J Consult Clin Psychol.* 2006 Feb;74(1):199-206.

58. Killaspy H, Bebbington P, Blizard R, et al. The REACT study: randomised evaluation of assertive community treatment in north London. *BMJ.* 2006;332(7545):815-20.

59. Gallo JJ, Bogner HR, Morales KH, Post EP, Lin JY, Bruce ML. The effect of a primary care practice-based depression intervention on mortality in older adults: a randomized trial.[Summary for patients in Ann Intern Med. 2007 May 15;146(10):I38; PMID: 17502628]. *Annals of Internal Medicine.* 2007;146(10):689-98.

60. Centers for Disease Control and Prevention (CDC). Suicide facts at a glance. *National Center for Injury Prevention and Control.* 2009; Available at http://www.cdc.gov/violenceprevention/pdf/Suicide-DataSheet-a.pdf. Accessed 1/3/2012.

61. Goldsmith SK, Pelmar TC, Kleinman AM, Bunny WE, eds. *Reducing suicide: A national imperative.* Washington (DC): National Academy Press; 2002.

62. Jordan JR. Is suicide bereavement different? A reassessment of the literature. *Suicide Life Threat Behav.* 2001;31(1):91-102.

63. Corso PS, Mercy JA, Simon TR, Finkelstein EA, Miller TR. Medical costs and productivity losses due to interpersonal and self-directed violence in the United States. *Am J Prev Med.* 2007 Jun;32(6):474-82.

64. Lambert MT. Seven-year outcomes of patients evaluated for suicidality. *Psychiatr Serv.* 2002;53(1):92-4.

65. Lambert MT, Fowler DR. Suicide risk factors among veterans: risk management in the changing culture of the Department of Veterans Affairs. *J Ment Health Adm.* 1997;24(3):350-8.

66. Martin J, Ghahramanlou-Holloway M, Lou K, Tucciarone P. A comparative review of U.S. Military and civilian suicide behavior: Implications for OEF/OIF suicide prevention efforts. *Journal of Mental Health and Counseling* 2009;31(2):101-18.

67. Schulberg HC, Bruce ML, Lee PW, Williams JWJ, Dietrich AJ. Preventing suicide in primary care patients: the primary care physician's role. *Gen Hosp Psychiatry.* 2004;26(5):337-45.

68. Teasdale T, Engberg A. Suicide after traumatic brain injury: a population study. *Journal of Neurology, Neurosurgery & Psychiatry.* 2001;71(4):436-40.

69. Joiner T. *Why people die by suicide.* Cambridge: Harvard University Press; 2005.

70. Brenner LA, Gutierrez PM, Cornette MM, Betthauser LM, Bahraini N, Staves PJ. A Qualitative study of potential suicide risk factors in returning combat veterans. *Journal of Mental Health Counseling.* 2008 Jul;30(3):211-25.

71. Cavanagh J, Carson A, Sharpe M, SM L. Psychological autopsy studies of suicide: A systematic review. *Psychological Medicine.* 2003;33:395-405.

72. Luoma J, Martin C, Pearson J. Contact with mental health and primary care providers before suicide: A review of the evidence. *American Journal of Psychiatry.* 2002;159(6):909-16.

73. Basham C, Denneson LM, Millet L, Shen X, Duckart J, Dobscha SK. Characteristics and VA Health Care Utilization of U. S. Veterans Who Completed Suicide in Oregon Between 2000 and 2005. *Suicide Life Threat Behav.* 2011 Apr 4;42(3):287-96.

74. Department of Veterans Affairs. 2001 National Survey of Veterans. 2001; Available at http://www.va.gov/VETDATA/docs/SurveysAndStudies/NSV_Final_Report.pdf. Accessed January 3, 2012.

75. Brown GK, Ten Have T, Henriques GR, Xie SX, Hollander JE, Beck AT. Cognitive therapy for the prevention of suicide attempts: a randomized controlled trial. *JAMA.* 2005 Aug 3;294(5):563-70.

76. Crawford MJ, Thomas O, Khan N, Kulinskaya E. Psychosocial interventions following self-harm: systematic review of their efficacy in preventing suicide. *Br J Psychiatry.* 2007 Jan;190:11-7.

77. Motto JA, Bostrom AG. A randomized controlled trial of postcrisis suicide prevention. *Psychiatr Serv.* 2001;52(6):828-33.

78. Paris J. Predicting and Preventing Suicide: Do We Know Enough to Do Either? *Harvard Review of Psychiatry.* 2006 Sep-Oct;14(5):233-40.

79. Moher D, Liberati A, Tetzlaff J, Altman DG, The Prisma Group. Preferred reporting items for systematic reviews and meta-analyses: the PRISMA statement. *PLoS Med.* 2009;6(7):e1000097.

80. Asenjo Lobos C, Komossa K, Rummel-Kluge C, et al. Clozapine versus other atypical antipsychotics for schizophrenia. *Cochrane Database Syst Rev.* 2010 (11):CD006633.

81. Barbui C, Furukawa TA, Cipriani A. Effectiveness of paroxetine in the treatment of acute major depression in adults: a systematic re-examination of published and unpublished data from randomized trials. *Canadian Medical Association Journal.* 2008;178(3):296-305.

82. Barbui C, Esposito E, Cipriani A. Selective serotonin reuptake inhibitors and risk of suicide: a systematic review of observational studies. *CMAJ.* 2009 Feb 3;180(3):291-7.

83. Cipriani A, Brambilla P, Furukawa T, et al. Fluoxetine versus other types of pharmacotherapy for depression. *Cochrane Database Syst Rev.* 2005 (4):CD004185.

84. Cipriani A, Pretty H, Hawton K, Geddes JR. Lithium in the prevention of suicidal behavior and all-cause mortality in patients with mood disorders: a systematic review of randomized trials. *Am J Psychiatry.* 2005 Oct;162(10):1805-19.

85. Cipriani A, Smith KA, Burgess SSA, Carney SM, Goodwin G, Geddes J. Lithium versus antidepressants in the long-term treatment of unipolar affective disorder. *Cochrane Database of Systematic Reviews.* 2009 (1).

86. Craig M, Howard L. Postnatal depression. *Clin Evid (Online).* 2009;2009.

87. Dubicka B, Elvins R, Roberts C, Chick G, Wilkinson P, Goodyer IM. Combined treatment with cognitive-behavioural therapy in adolescent depression: meta-analysis. *Br J Psychiatry.* 2010 Dec;197:433-40.

88. Grandjean EM, Aubry JM. Lithium: updated human knowledge using an evidence-based approach: Part I: Clinical efficacy in bipolar disorder. *CNS Drugs.* 2009;23(3):225-40.

89. Hazell P. Depression in children and adolescents. *Clin Evid (Online).* 2011;2011.

90.   Innamorati M, Pompili M, Amore M, et al. Suicide prevention in late life: Is there sound evidence for practice? In: Pompili M, Tatarelli R, eds. *Evidence-based practice in suicidology: A source book.* Cambridge, MA: Hogrefe Publishing; 2011:211-32.

91.   Hammerness PG, Vivas FM, Geller DA. Selective serotonin reuptake inhibitors in pediatric psychopharmacology: a review of the evidence. *J Pediatr.* 2006 Feb;148(2):158-65.

92.   McDonagh M, Peterson K, Carson S, Fu R, Thakurta S. Drug Class Review: Atypical Antipsychotic Drugs: Final Update 3 Report. *Drug Effectiveness Review Project.* 2010 Jul:Oregon Health and Science University.

93.   Robinson J, Hetrick SE, Martin C. Preventing suicide in young people: systematic review. *Aust N Z J Psychiatry.* 2011 Jan;45(1):3-26.

94.   Sakinofsky I. Treating suicidality in depressive illness. Part 2: does treatment cure or cause suicidality? *Can J Psychiatry.* 2007 Jun;52(6 Suppl 1):85S-101S.

95.   Sakinofsky I. Treating suicidality in depressive illness. Part 1: current controversies. *Can J Psychiatry.* 2007 Jun;52(6 Suppl 1):71S-84S.

96.   Soomro GM. Deliberate self-harm (and attempted suicide). *Clin Evid (Online).* 2008;12:1012.

97.   Van Lieshout RJ, MacQueen GM. Efficacy and acceptability of mood stabilisers in the treatment of acute bipolar depression: systematic review. *Br J Psychiatry.* 2010 Apr;196:266-73.

98.   Williams SB, O'Connor E, Eder M, Whitlock E. Screening for Child and Adolescent Depression In Primary Care Settings: A Systematic Evidence Review for the U.S. Preventive Services Task Force. 2009 Apr.

99.   Williams SB, O'Connor EA, Eder M, Whitlock EP. Screening for child and adolescent depression in primary care settings: a systematic evidence review for the US Preventive Services Task Force. *Pediatrics.* 2009 Apr;123(4):e716-35.

100.   National Collaborating Centre for Mental Health. Depression in children and young people: identification and management in primary, community and secondary care. *British Psychological Society.* 2005:233.

101.   Ziemba KS, O'Carroll CB, Drazkowski JF, et al. Do antiepileptic drugs increase the risk of suicidality in adult patients with epilepsy?: a critically appraised topic. *Neurologist.* 2010 Sep;16(5):325-8.

102.   Abbass AA, Hancock JT, Henderson J, Kisely SR. Short-term psychodynamic psychotherapies for common mental disorders. *Cochrane Database of Systematic Reviews.* 2009 (1).

103.   Bagley SC, Munjas B, Shekelle P. A systematic review of suicide prevention programs for military or veterans. *Suicide Life Threat Behav.* 2010 Jun;40(3):257-65.

104. Binks C, Fenton M, McCarthy L, Lee T, Adams CE, Duggan C. Psychological therapies for people with borderline personality disorder. *Cochrane Database of Systematic Reviews.* 2011 (1).

105. Corcoran J, Dattalo P, Crowley M, Brown E, Grindle L. A systematic review of psychosocial interventions for suicidal adolescents. *Children and Youth Services Review.* 2011 Nov;33(11):2112-8.

106. Dieterich M, Irving CB, Park B, Marshall M. Intensive case management for severe mental illness. *Cochrane Database Syst Rev.* 2010 (10):CD007906.

107. Irving C, B., Adams CE, Rice K. Crisis intervention for people with severe mental illnesses. *Cochrane Database of Systematic Reviews.* 2010 (5).

108. Kavanagh J, Oliver S, Caird J, et al. Inequalities and the mental health of young people: a systematic review of secondary school-based cognitive behavioural interventions (Structured abstract). *University of London, Institute of Education, Social Science Research Unit, EPPI-Centre.* 2009:1-109.

109. Lapierre S, Erlangsen A, Waern M, et al. A systematic review of elderly suicide prevention programs. *Crisis.* 2011 Jan 1;32(2):88-98.

110. Leenaars AA. Evidence-based psychotherapy with suicidal people: A systematic review. *Pompili, Maurizio [Ed].* 2011:89-123.

111. Muralidharan S, Fenton M. Containment strategies for people with serious mental illness. *Cochrane Database of Systematic Reviews.* 2009 (1).

112. Newton AS, Hamm MP, Bethell J, et al. Pediatric suicide-related presentations: a systematic review of mental health care in the emergency department. *Ann Emerg Med.* 2010 Dec;56(6):649-59.

113. Pharoah F, Mari J, Rathbone J, Wong W. Family intervention for schizophrenia. *Cochrane Database Syst Rev.* 2010 (12):CD000088.

114. Shek E, Stein A, T., Shansis FM, Marshall M, Crowther R, Tyrer P. Day hospital versus outpatient care for people with schizophrenia. *Cochrane Database of Systematic Reviews.* 2010 (11).

115. State of Victoria Department of Health. Suicide risk assessment and management: A systematic evidence review for the Clinical practice guidelines for emergency departments and mental health services project. *Mental Health, Drugs and Regions Division.* 2010.

116. Takada M, Shima S. Characteristics and effects of suicide prevention programs: comparison between workplace and other settings. *Ind Health.* 2010;48(4):416-26.

117. Bateman A, Fonagy P. 8-year follow-up of patients treated for borderline personality disorder: mentalization-based treatment versus treatment as usual. *The American Journal of Psychiatry.* 2008 May;165(5):631-8.

118.   Hailey D, Roine R, Ohinmaa A. The effectiveness of telemental health applications: A review. *The Canadian Journal of Psychiatry / La Revue canadienne de psychiatrie.* 2008 Nov;53(11):769-78.

119.   van der Feltz-Cornelis CM, Sarchiapone M, Postuvan V, et al. Best Practice Elements of Multilevel Suicide Prevention Strategies. *Crisis.* 2011 Sep 26:1-15.

120.   Bruce M, Ten Have T, Reynolds CI, et al. Reducing suicidal ideation and depressive symptoms in depressed older primary care patients: a randomized controlled trial. *JAMA.* 2004;291(9):1081-91.

121.   Wortzel HS, Gutierrez PM, Homaifar BY, Breshears RE, Harwood JE. Surrogate endpoints in suicide research. *Suicide Life Threat Behav.* 2010 Oct;40(5):500-5.

122.   Wasserman D, Wasserman C, eds. *Oxford Textbook of Suicidology and Suicide Prevention: A Global Perspective.* New York: Oxford University Press; 2009.

123.   Shekelle P, Woolf S, Eccles M, Grimshaw J. Clinical guidelines: Developing guidelines. *British Medical Journal.* 1999;318(7183):593-6.

124.   Vitiello B, Silva SG, Rohde P, et al. Suicidal events in the Treatment for Adolescents With Depression Study (TADS). *J Clin Psychiatry.* 2009 May;70(5):741-7.

125.   March J, Silva S, Vitiello B, Team T. The Treatment for Adolescents with Depression Study (TADS): methods and message at 12 weeks. *Journal of the American Academy of Child and Adolescent Psychiatry.* 2006 Dec;45(12):1393-403.

126.   Brent D, Emslie G, Clarke G, et al. Switching to another SSRI or to venlafaxine with or without cognitive behavioral therapy for adolescents with SSRI-resistant depression: the TORDIA randomized controlled trial. *JAMA.* 2008;299(8):901-13.

127.   Schulberg HC, Bryce C, Chism K, et al. Managing late-life depression in primary care practice: a case study of the Health Specialist's role. *International Journal of Geriatric Psychiatry.* 2001;16(6):577-84.

128.   Bogner HR, Morales KH, Post EP, Bruce ML. Diabetes, depression, and death: a randomized controlled trial of a depression treatment program for older adults based in primary care (PROSPECT). *Diabetes Care.* 2007 Dec;30(12):3005-10.

129.   Raue PJ, Morales KH, Post EP, Bogner HR, Have TT, Bruce ML. The wish to die and 5-year mortality in elderly primary care patients. *Am J Geriatr Psychiatry.* 2010 Apr;18(4):341-50.

APPENDIX A. SEARCH STRATEGIES

PubMed searched from 2005 – November 18, 2011	
Suicide	"Suicide"[Mesh] OR "Suicide, Attempted"[Mesh] OR suicid*
Risk	"Risk"[Mesh] OR "Risk Assessment"[Mesh] OR "Risk Factors"[Mesh] OR risk[Title/Abstract]
Screening	"mass screening"[Mesh] OR "Validation studies"[Publication Type] OR Screening[title] OR screen[title] OR assessment[title] OR assessments[title] OR questionnaire[title] OR questionnaires[title] OR instrument[title] OR instruments[title] OR tool[title] OR tools[title] OR scale[title] OR scales[title] OR measure[title] OR measures[title]
Prevention	Prevent* OR depression OR health education OR health promotion OR public opinion OR mass screening OR family physicians OR medical Education OR primary healthcare OR antidepressive agents OR psychotherapy OR schools OR adolescents OR methods OR firearms OR overdose OR poisoning OR gas poisoning OR mass media
Suicide Prevention	("Suicide/prevention and control"[Mesh] OR Suicide, Attempted/ prevention and contril"[Mesh]) NOT (case report* OR editorial* OR letter)
Suicide Prevention OR (Suicide AND (Risk OR Screening OR Prevention)	

PsycINFO, Cochrane and HAPI Search November 18, 2011

Limited from 2005 – November 18, 2011

Search Strategy:

----

1 exp Attempted Suicide/ or exp Suicide Prevention/

2 (prevent* or depression or health education or health promotion or public opinion or mass screening or family physicians or medical education or primary health care or antidepressive agents or psychotherapy or schools or adolescents or methods or firearms or overdose or poisoning or gas poisoning or mass media).mp. [mp=title, abstract, heading word, table of contents, key concepts, original title, tests & measures]

3 suicide.mp. [mp=title, abstract, heading word, table of contents, key concepts, original title, tests & measures]

4 2 and 3

5 1 or 4

6 exp Case Report/

7 editorial.mp.

8 letter.mp.

9   6 or 7 or 8

10   5 not 9

11   exp Attempted Suicide/ or exp Suicide/ or suicide.mp.

12   (suicide or suicidal or suicides or sucidality).mp. [mp=title, abstract, heading word, table of contents, key concepts, original title, tests & measures]

13   11 or 12

14   exp Risk Assessment/ or risk.mp. or exp Risk Factors/

15   exp Screening/

16   exp test validity/

17   screening.m_titl.

18   screen.m_titl.

19   assessment.m_titl.

20   assessments.m_titl.

21   questionnaire.m_titl.

22   questionnaires.m_titl.

23   instrument.m_titl.

24   instruments.m_titl.

25   tool.m_titl.

26   tools.m_titl.

27   scales.m_titl.

28   measure.m_titl.

29   measures.m_titl.

30   risk.mp.

31   14 or 15 or 16 or 17 or 18 or 19 or 20 or 21 or 22 or 23 or 24 or 25 or 26 or 27 or 28 or 29 or 30

32   13 and 31

33   10 or 32

APPENDIX B. STUDY SELECTION FORM

VA ESP Suicide Prevention Study Selection Process: Coding

Step 1: Importing citations

- Enter database name, search date, and other details into Custom 1.

Step 2: Title/Abstract level coding

- The objective of the title/abstract review phase is to eliminate obviously irrelevant publications. Abstracts that lack an explicit reference to suicidal self-directed violence (e.g., suicidality, behaviors, attempts, and suicides) will be excluded at this phase. Reviewers will provide decision and characteristic codes and these will be recorded in Custom 3 of the EndNote library.
  - Decision codes:
    - **R**=Retrieve
    - **E**=Exclude
    - **B**=Retrieve for Background
  - Characteristic codes: Our first priority is retrieval of systematic reviews, especially those focusing on Veteran/military populations. Our second priority is retrieval of primary studies in Veteran/military populations. For ease of identifying these subsets of publications in the ENL, reviewers should add either or both of the following codes when applicable:
    - **SR**=systematic review
    - **V**=Veteran and/or military population

Step 3: Full-text level coding

- Record final decision to include study in review, and any other study characteristics of interest.
  - **Characteristics of interest (recorded in Custom Fields):**
    - Population: Veteran/Military or Non-Veteran/Military
    - Intervention Type: Psychotherapy, Pharmacotherapy, or Referral/Follow-up
    - Study Design: Systematic Review, clinical trial (randomized or nonrandomized), observational study, other
  - **Full-text exclusion codes to be entered into Custom 4:**
    - 1=Non-English language
    - 2=Ineligible country (only including US, UK, Canada, New Zealand, Australia)
    - 3=Ineligible outcome
    - 4=Ineligible intervention (i.e., broadly focused public health interventions implemented among populations, etc.)
    - 5=Study does not evaluate interventions
    - 6=Ineligible publication type (e.g., letter, editorial, publication available only as abstract, non-systematic review, etc.)
    - 7=Ineligible systematic review due to limitations in quality
    - 8=Nonsystematic regulatory agency analysis

- 9=Non-RCT study design

- Full-text coding to be completed in the format of a label affixed to each publication in the format shown below. Reviewer 1 will circle relevant characteristics and inclusion decision, and list an exclusion code when applicable. Reviewer 2 will verify Reviewer 1's decisions and circle Agree or Disagree. All disagreements will be resolved using a consensus process and consensus decisions recorded.

Pop: Vet-Mil / Non-Vet-Mil
Intervention: Meds / Thpy / Ref-FU / NA
Design: SR / CT / Obs / Other
Rev1: Include / Exclude – Code: _____
Rev2: Agree / Disagree Consensus: _____

APPENDIX C. CRITERIA USED IN QUALITY ASSESSMENT OF SYSTEMATIC REVIEWS

Criteria	Operationalization of Criteria*
1. Were the search methods reported? *Were the search methods used to find evidence (original research) on the primary questions stated?* "Yes" if the review states the databases used, date of most recent searches, and some mention of search terms.	The purpose of this index is to evaluate the scientific quality (i.e., adherence to scientific principles) of research overviews (review articles) published in the medical literature. It is not intended to measure literary quality, importance, relevance, originality, or other attributes of overviews.
2. Was the search comprehensive? *Was the search for evidence reasonably comprehensive?* "Yes" if the review searches at least 2 databases and looks at other sources (such as reference lists, hand searches, queries experts).	The index is for assessing overviews of primary ("original") research on pragmatic questions regarding causation, diagnosis, prognosis, therapy, or prevention. A research overview is a survey of research. The same principles that apply to epidemiological surveys apply to overviews: a question must be clearly specified, a target population identified and accessed; appropriate information obtained from that population in an unbiased fashion; and conclusions derived, sometimes with the help of formal statistical analysis, as is done in "meta-analyses". The fundamental difference between overviews and epidemiological studies is the unit of analysis, not the scientific issues that the questions in this index address.
3. Were the inclusion criteria reported? *Were the criteria used for deciding which studies to include in the overview reported?*	
4. Was selection bias avoided? *Was bias in the selection of studies avoided?* "Yes" if the review reports how many studies were identified by searches, numbers excluded, and gives appropriate reasons for excluding them (usually because of pre-defined inclusion/exclusion criteria).	Since most published overviews do not include a methods section, it is difficult to answer some of the questions in the index. Base your answers, as much as possible, on information provided in the overview. If the methods that were used are reported incompletely relative to a specific question, score it as "can't tell," unless there is information in the overview to suggest either the criterion was or was not met.
5. Were the validity criteria reported? *Were the criteria used for assessing the validity of the included studies reported?*	
6. Was validity assessed appropriately? *Was the validity of all the studies referred to in the text assessed using appropriate criteria (either in selecting studies for inclusion or in analyzing the studies that are cited)?* "Yes" if the review reports validity assessment and did some type of analysis with it (e.g., sensitivity analysis of results according to quality ratings, excluded low-quality studies, etc.)	
7. Were the methods used to combine studies reported? *Were the methods used to combine the findings of the relevant studies (to reach a conclusion) reported?* "Yes" for studies that did qualitative analysis if there is some mention that quantitative analysis was not possible and reasons that it could not be done, or if 'best evidence' or some other grading of evidence scheme used.	
8. Were the findings combined appropriately? *Were the findings of the relevant studies combined appropriately relative to the primary question the overview addresses?* "Yes" if the review performs a test for heterogeneity before pooling, does appropriate subgroup testing, appropriate sensitivity analysis, or other such analysis.	For Question 8, if no attempt has been made to combine findings, and no statement is made regarding the inappropriateness of combining findings, check "No" if a summary (general) estimate is given anywhere in the abstract, the discussion, or the summary section of the paper; and if it is not reported how that estimate was derived, mark "No" even if there is a statement regarding the limitations of combining the findings of the studies reviewed. If in doubt, mark "Can't tell".
9. Were the conclusions supported by the reported data? *Were the conclusions made by the author(s) supported by the data and/or analysis reported in the overview?*	For an overview to be scored as "Yes" in Question 9, data (not just citations) must be reported that support the main conclusions regarding the primary question(s) that the overview addresses.
10. What was the overall scientific quality of the overview? *How would you rate the scientific quality of this overview?*	The score for Question 10, the overall scientific quality, should be based on your answers to the first nine questions. The following guidelines can be used to assist with deriving a summary score: If the "Can't tell" option is used one or more times on the preceding questions, a review is likely to have minor flaws at best and it is difficult to rule out major flaws (i.e., a score of 4 or lower). If the "No" option is used on Question 2, 4, 6 or 8, the review is likely to have major flaws (i.e., a score of 3 or less, depending on the number and degree of the flaws).

Scoring

Extensive Flaws	Major Flaws			Minor Flaws		Minimal Flaws
1	2	3	4	5	6	7

Each Question is scored as Yes, Partially/Can't tell or No

*Table created using information from Oxman & Guyatt, *J Clin Epidemiol.* 1991;44(11):1271-8 and Furlan, Clarke, et al. *Spine.* 2001 Apr 1;26(7):E155-62.

APPENDIX D. CRITERIA USED IN QUALITY ASSESSMENT OF RANDOMIZED CONTROLLED TRIALS[16]

The Cochrane Collaboration's tool for assessing risk of bias[16]

Domain	Description	Review authors' judgment
Sequence generation	Describe the method used to generate the allocation sequence in sufficient detail to allow an assessment of whether it should produce comparable groups.	Was the allocation sequence adequately generated?
Allocation concealment	Describe the method used to conceal the allocation sequence in sufficient detail to determine whether intervention allocations could have been foreseen in advance of or during enrollment.	Was allocation adequately concealed?
Blinding of participants, personnel and outcome assessors *Assessments should be made for each main outcome (or class of outcomes)*	Describe all measures used, if any, to blind study participants and personnel from knowledge of which intervention a participant received. Provide any information relating to whether the intended blinding was effective.	Was knowledge of the allocated intervention adequately prevented during the study?
Incomplete outcome data *Assessments should be made for each main outcome (or class of outcomes)*	Describe the completeness of outcome data for each main outcome, including attrition and exclusions from the analysis. State whether attrition and exclusions were reported, the numbers in each intervention group (compared with total randomized participants), reasons for attrition/exclusions where reported, and any re-inclusions in analyses performed by the review authors.	Were incomplete outcome data adequately addressed?
Selective outcome reporting	State how the possibility of selective outcome reporting was examined by the review authors, and what was found.	Are reports of the study free of suggestion of selective outcome reporting?
Other sources of bias	State any important concerns about bias not addressed in the other domains in the tool. If particular questions/entries were pre-specified in the review's protocol, responses should be provided for each question/entry.	Was the study apparently free of other problems that could put it at a high risk of bias?

Possible approach for *summary assessments* outcome (across domains) within and across studies

Risk of bias	Interpretation	Within a study	Across studies
Low risk of bias	Plausible bias unlikely to seriously alter the results.	Low risk of bias for all key domains.	Most information is from studies at low risk of bias.
Unclear risk of bias	Plausible bias that raises some doubt about the results.	Unclear risk of bias for one or more key domains.	Most information is from studies at low or unclear risk of bias.
High risk of bias	Plausible bias that seriously weakens confidence in the results.	High risk of bias for one or more key domains.	The proportion of information from studies at high risk of bias is sufficient to affect the interpretation of the results.

Criteria for judging risk of bias in the 'Risk of bias' assessment tool

SEQUENCE GENERATION
Was the allocation sequence adequately generated? [Short form: *Adequate sequence generation?*]

Criteria for a judgment of 'YES' (i.e., low risk of bias)	The investigators describe a random component in the sequence generation process such as: ▪ Referring to a random number table; using a computer random number generator; coin tossing; shuffling cards or envelopes; throwing dice; drawing of lots; minimization.* *Minimization may be implemented without a random element, and this is considered to be equivalent to being random.
Criteria for the judgment of 'NO' (i.e., high risk of bias)	The investigators describe a non-random component in the sequence generation process. Usually, the description would involve some systematic, non-random approach, for example: ▪ Sequence generated by odd or even date of birth; ▪ Sequence generated by some rule based on date (or day) of admission; ▪ Sequence generated by some rule based on hospital or clinic record number. Other non-random approaches happen much less frequently than the systematic approaches mentioned above and tend to be obvious. They usually involve judgment or some method of non-random categorization of participants, for example: ▪ Allocation by judgment of the clinician; ▪ Allocation by preference of the participant; ▪ Allocation based on the results of a laboratory test or a series of tests; ▪ Allocation by availability of the intervention.
Criteria for the judgment of 'UNCLEAR' (uncertain risk of bias)	Insufficient information about the sequence generation process to permit judgment of 'Yes' or 'No'.

ALLOCATION CONCEALMENT
Was allocation adequately concealed? [Short form: *Allocation concealment?*]

Criteria for a judgment of 'YES' (i.e., low risk of bias)	Participants and investigators enrolling participants could not foresee assignment because one of the following, or an equivalent method, was used to conceal allocation: ▪ Central allocation (including telephone, web-based, and pharmacy-controlled randomization); ▪ Sequentially numbered drug containers of identical appearance; ▪ Sequentially numbered, opaque, sealed envelopes.
Criteria for the judgment of 'NO' (i.e., high risk of bias)	Participants or investigators enrolling participants could possibly foresee assignments and thus introduce selection bias, such as allocation based on: ▪ Using an open random allocation schedule (e.g., a list of random numbers); ▪ Assignment envelopes were used without appropriate safeguards (e.g., if envelopes were unsealed or non-opaque or not sequentially numbered); ▪ Alternation or rotation; ▪ Date of birth; ▪ Case record number; ▪ Any other explicitly unconcealed procedure.
Criteria for the judgment of 'UNCLEAR' (uncertain risk of bias)	Insufficient information to permit judgment of 'Yes' or 'No'. This is usually the case if the method of concealment is not described or not described in sufficient detail to allow a definite judgment – for example, if the use of assignment envelopes is described, but it remains unclear whether envelopes were sequentially numbered, opaque and sealed.

BLINDING OF PARTICIPANTS, PERSONNEL AND OUTCOME ASSESSORS
Was knowledge of the allocated interventions adequately prevented during the study? [Short form: *Blinding?*]

Criteria for a judgment of 'YES' (i.e., low risk of bias)	Any one of the following: ■ No blinding, but the review authors judge that the outcome and the outcome measurement are not likely to be influenced by lack of blinding; ■ Blinding of participants and key study personnel ensured, and unlikely that the blinding could have been broken; ■ Either participants or some key study personnel were not blinded, but outcome assessment was blinded and the non-blinding of others unlikely to introduce bias.
Criteria for the judgment of 'NO' (i.e., high risk of bias)	Any one of the following: ■ No blinding or incomplete blinding, and the outcome or outcome measurement is likely to be influenced by lack of blinding; ■ Blinding of key study participants and personnel attempted, but likely that the blinding could have been broken; ■ Either participants or some key study personnel were not blinded, and the non-blinding of others likely to introduce bias.
Criteria for the judgment of 'UNCLEAR' (uncertain risk of bias)	Any one of the following: ■ Insufficient information to permit judgment of 'Yes' or 'No'; ■ The study did not address this outcome.

INCOMPLETE OUTCOME DATA
Were incomplete outcome data adequately addressed? [Short form: *Incomplete outcome data addressed?*]

Criteria for a judgment of 'YES' (i.e., low risk of bias)	Any one of the following: ■ No missing outcome data; ■ Reasons for missing outcome data unlikely to be related to true outcome (for survival data, censoring unlikely to be introducing bias); ■ Missing outcome data balanced in numbers across intervention groups, with similar reasons for missing data across groups; ■ For dichotomous outcome data, the proportion of missing outcomes compared with observed event risk not enough to have a clinically relevant impact on the intervention effect estimate; ■ For continuous outcome data, plausible effect size (difference in means or standardized difference in means) among missing outcomes not enough to have a clinically relevant impact on observed effect size; ■ Missing data have been imputed using appropriate methods.
Criteria for the judgment of 'NO' (i.e., high risk of bias)	Any one of the following: ■ Reason for missing outcome data likely to be related to true outcome, with either imbalance in numbers or reasons for missing data across intervention groups; ■ For dichotomous outcome data, the proportion of missing outcomes compared with observed event risk enough to induce clinically relevant bias in intervention effect estimate; ■ For continuous outcome data, plausible effect size (difference in means or standardized difference in means) among missing outcomes enough to induce clinically relevant bias in observed effect size; ■ 'As-treated' analysis done with substantial departure of the intervention received from that assigned at randomization; ■ Potentially inappropriate application of simple imputation.
Criteria for the judgment of 'UNCLEAR' (uncertain risk of bias)	Any one of the following: ■ Insufficient reporting of attrition/exclusions to permit judgment of 'Yes' or 'No' (e.g., number randomized not stated, no reasons for missing data provided); ■ The study did not address this outcome.

SELECTIVE OUTCOME REPORTING
Are reports of the study free of suggestion of selective outcome reporting? [Short form: *Free of selective reporting?*]

Criteria for a judgment of 'YES' (i.e., low risk of bias)	Any of the following: ▪ The study protocol is available and all of the study's pre-specified (primary and secondary) outcomes that are of interest in the review have been reported in the pre-specified way; ▪ The study protocol is not available but it is clear that the published reports include all expected outcomes, including those that were pre-specified (convincing text of this nature may be uncommon).
Criteria for the judgment of 'NO' (i.e., high risk of bias)	Any one of the following: ▪ Not all of the study's pre-specified primary outcomes have been reported; ▪ One or more primary outcomes is reported using measurements, analysis methods or subsets of the data (e.g., subscales) that were not pre-specified; ▪ One or more reported primary outcomes were not pre-specified (unless clear justification for their reporting is provided, such as an unexpected adverse effect); ▪ One or more outcomes of interest in the review are reported incompletely so that they cannot be entered in a meta-analysis; ▪ The study report fails to include results for a key outcome that would be expected to have been reported for such a study.
Criteria for the judgment of 'UNCLEAR' (uncertain risk of bias)	Insufficient information to permit judgment of 'Yes' or 'No'. It is likely that the majority of studies will fall into this category.

OTHER POTENTIAL THREATS TO VALIDITY

Was the study apparently free of other problems that could put it at a risk of bias? [Short form: *Free of other bias*?]

Criteria for a judgment of 'YES' (i.e., low risk of bias)	The study appears to be free of other sources of bias.
Criteria for the judgment of 'NO' (i.e., high risk of bias)	There is at least one important risk of bias. For example, the study: ▪ Had a potential source of bias related to the specific study design used; or ▪ Stopped early due to some data-dependent process (including a formal-stopping rule); or ▪ Had extreme baseline imbalance; or ▪ Has been claimed to have been fraudulent; or ▪ Had some other problem.
Criteria for the judgment of 'UNCLEAR' (uncertain risk of bias)	There may be a risk of bias, but there is either: ▪ Insufficient information to assess whether an important risk of bias exists; or ▪ Insufficient rationale or evidence that an identified problem will introduce bias.

APPENDIX E. CRITERIA USED TO ASSESS STRENGTH OF EVIDENCE[17]

Definitions of the Grades of Overall Strength of Evidence

Grade	Definition
High	High confidence that the evidence reflects the true effect. Further research is very unlikely to change our confidence in the estimate of effect.
Moderate	Moderate confidence that the evidence reflects the true effect. Further research may change our confidence in the estimate of the effect and may change the estimate.
Low	Low confidence that the evidence reflects the true effect. Further research is likely to change our confidence in the estimate of the effect and is likely to change the estimate.
Insufficient	Evidence either is unavailable or does not permit estimation of an effect.

Domains Used to Grade the Strength of Evidence

Domain	Definition and Elements	Score and Application
Risk of bias	Risk of bias is the degree to which the included studies for a given outcome or comparison have a high likelihood of adequate protection against bias (i.e., good internal validity), assessed through two main elements: • Study design (e.g., RCTs or observational studies) • Aggregate quality of the studies under consideration. Information for this determination comes from the rating of quality (good/fair/poor) done for individual studies.	Use one of the three levels of aggregate risk of bias: • Low risk of bias • Medium risk of bias • High risk of bias
Consistency	The principle definition of consistency is the degree to which reported effect sizes from included studies appear to have the same direction of effect. This can be assessed through two main elements: • Effect sizes have the same sign (that is, are on the same side of "no effect"). • The range of effect sizes is narrow.	Use one of the three levels of consistency: • Consistent (i.e., no inconsistency) • Inconsistent • Unknown or not applicable (e.g., single study) As noted in the text, single-study evidence bases (even mega trials) cannot be judged with respect to consistency. In that instance, use "Consistency unknown (single study)".

Directness	The rating of directness relates to whether the evidence links the interventions directly to health outcomes. For a comparison of two treatments, directness implies that head-to-head trials measure the most important health or ultimate outcomes. Two types of indirectness, which can coexist, may be of concern. Evidence is indirect if: • It uses intermediate or surrogate outcomes instead of ultimate health outcomes. In this case, one body of evidence links the intervention to intermediate outcomes and another body of evidence links the intermediate to most important (health or ultimate) outcomes. • It uses two or more bodies of evidence to compare interventions A and B – e.g., studies of A vs. placebo and B vs. placebo, or studies of A vs. C and B vs. C but not A vs. B. Indirectness always implies that more than one body of evidence is required to link interventions to the most important health outcomes. Directness may be contingent on the outcomes of interest. EPC authors are expected to make clear the outcomes involved when assessing this domain.	Score dichotomously as one of two levels directness: • Direct • Indirect If indirect, specify which of the two types of indirectness accounts for the rating (or both, if that is the case) – namely, use of intermediate/ surrogate outcomes rather than health outcomes, and use of indirect comparisons. Comment on the potential weaknesses caused by, or inherent in, the indirect analysis. The EPC should note if both direct and indirect evidence was available, particularly when indirect evidence supports a small body of direct evidence.
Precision	Precision is the degree of certainty surrounding an effect estimate with respect to a given outcome (i.e., for each outcome separately). If a meta-analysis was performed, this will be the CI around the summary effect size.	Score dichotomously as one of two levels of precision: • Precise • Imprecise A precise estimate is an estimate that would allow a clinically useful conclusion. An imprecise estimate is one for which the CI is wide enough to include clinically distinct conclusions. For example, results may be statistically compatible with both clinically important superiority and inferiority (i.e., the direction of effect is unknown), a circumstance that will preclude a valid conclusion.
Strength of association (magnitude of effect)	Strength of association refers to the likelihood that the observed effect is large enough that it cannot have occurred solely as a result of bias from potential confounding factors.	This additional domain should be considered if the effect size is particularly large. Use one of two levels: • Strong: large effect size that is unlikely to have occurred in the absence of a true effect of the intervention. • Weak: small enough effect size that it could have occurred solely as a result of bias from confounding factors.

APPENDIX F. QUALITY RATING OF SYSTEMATIC REVIEWS RELATED TO PHARMACOTHERAPY USING OXMAN AND GUYATT[15] CRITERIA

Author Year of systematic review	Search methods reported	Comprehensive search	Inclusion criteria reported	Selection bias avoided	Validity criteria reported	Validity assessed appropriately	Methods used to combine studies reported	Findings combined appropriately	Conclusions supported by data	Overall scientific quality (higher score is better)
Asenjo Lobos 2010[80]	Yes	Yes	Yes	Yes	Yes	Yes; excluded studies where sequence generation was at high risk of bias or where allocation was clearly not concealed.	Yes	Yes	Yes	7
Barbui 2008[81]	Yes	Yes	Yes	Yes	Yes	Yes	Yes	Yes	Yes	7
Barbui 2009[82]	Yes	Yes	Yes	Yes	Yes	Yes	Yes	Yes	Yes	7
Cipriani 2005 (Fluoxetine)[83]	Yes	Yes	Yes	Yes	Yes	Yes; no variation to analyze.	Yes	Can't tell for suicide; reported no differences between fluoxetine and control AD among 4 studies but analysis of heterogeneity not reported.	Yes	6
Cipriani 2005 (Lithium)[84]	Yes	Yes	Yes	Yes; study flow diagram provided reasons for exclusion.	Yes	No; reported allocation concealment, blinding and ITT analysis; no analysis based on quality, despite some variation in use of blinding.	Yes	Yes	Yes	6
Cipriani 2009[85]	Yes	Yes	Yes	Yes	Yes	Yes; those rated C (inadequate) excluded from analysis.	Yes	Yes	Yes	7
Craig 2009[86]	No; no mention of search terms.	No; no supplemental sources.	Yes	No; detailed results of study selection not reported, no reasons for exclusions described.	No	Can't tell; within GRADE evaluation of quality of evidence, deducted points for internal validity limitations; but, unclear as to the scope of the internal validity domains assessed.	Yes	Yes	Yes	3

Suicide Prevention Interventions and Referral/Follow-up Services: A Systematic Review

Author Year of systematic review	Search methods reported	Comprehensive search	Inclusion criteria reported	Selection bias avoided	Validity criteria reported	Validity assessed appropriately	Methods used to combine studies reported	Findings combined appropriately	Conclusions supported by data	Overall scientific quality (higher score is better)
Dubicka 2010[87]	Yes	Yes	Yes	Yes; study flow diagram provided reasons for exclusion.	Yes	Yes; reported results of validity assessment; none were poor, not necessarily a need to control for variation in synthesis.	Yes	Yes	Yes	7
Grandjean 2009[88]	Yes	No; only one database.	No	Can't tell.	No	Can't tell; validity of all studies not provided, but noted that only publications with the highest standards of quality were selected.	No	Can't tell; methods not reported.	Yes	2
Hammerness 2006[91]	Yes	No; only one database.	No	Can't tell; numbers and reasons for exclusions not reported.	Yes	Can't tell; validity of studies not referred to in text.	Can't tell; no mention of consideration of quantitative analysis and no grading of strength of evidence.	Yes	Yes	5
Hazell 2011[89]	Partially; no mention of search terms	No; no supplemental sources.	Yes	Can't tell; numbers and reasons for exclusions not reported	No	Yes; validity assessment included in GRADE strength of evidence ratings.	Yes; used GRADE approach to rate strength of evidence.	Yes	Yes	5
Innamorati 2011[90]	Yes	No; no supplemental sources.	No; no information on PICOTS.	Can't tell; only reported number of included studies.	No; none described; only use of Shekelle 1999[123] scheme for classifying study design and strength of recommendation, but no quality.	No	Yes; used Shekelle 1999[123] scheme for classifying study design and strength of recommendation.	Yes	Yes	3
McDonagh 2010[92]	Yes	Yes	Yes	Yes	Yes	Yes	Yes	Yes	Yes	7
National Collaborating Centre for Mental Health 2005[100]	Yes	Yes	Yes	Yes	Yes	Yes	Yes	Yes	Yes	7

Author Year of systematic review	Search methods reported	Comprehensive search	Inclusion criteria reported	Selection bias avoided	Validity criteria reported	Validity assessed appropriately	Methods used to combine studies reported	Findings combined appropriately	Conclusions supported by data	Overall scientific quality (higher score is better)
Robinson 2011[93]	Yes	Yes	Yes	Can't tell; numbers of exclusions reported at each stage, but reasons not reported.	Yes	No; reported results of validity assessment in table and paragraph, but did not appear to account for variation in synthesis.	Yes	No; only 1 comparison with >1 study and did not combine data and did not explain reasons for this.	Yes	4
Sakinofsky 2007 (Parts 1 & 2)[94,95]	Partially; start date provided, but no end date.	Yes; several databases were used.	Can't tell; RCTs were the main focus but of necessity, it also considered other categories of investigations of the outcome of treatment.	No; no information related to number of articles found, included, and excluded.	No; did not describe criteria used to differentiate between good and deficiencies.	Yes; critical assessment of the quality of design, conduct and analysis of the studies was performed and reported according to authors' constructed schema of level of evidence.	Yes	Yes; report of findings follow simplified scheme of evidence constructed by authors.	Yes	4
Soomro 2008[96]	Yes	No; no hand-searching, reference list searching, or asking experts noted.	Yes	No	Yes	Yes	No	Yes	Yes	4
Van Lieshout 2010[97]	Yes	Yes	Yes	Yes; study flow diagram provided reasons for exclusion.	Yes	Yes; only included studies with a Jadad score of ≥3.	Yes; used GRADE approach to rate strength of evidence.	Yes; no significant heterogeneity reported.	Yes	7
Williams 2009[98] & Williams 2009[99]	Yes	Yes	Yes	Yes; study flow diagram in Pediatrics publication,[99] reasons for exclusion for individual trials provided in Evidence Report.[98]	Yes	Yes; excluded poor quality studies.	Yes	Yes; did not conduct meta-analyses due to heterogeneity.	Yes	7
Ziemba 2010[101]	Yes	Yes; searched references lists which led to identification of FDA meta-analysis.	No	No; not reported.	No	Can't tell; only reported one study, described as the highest level of evidence they found.	No	No; methods not reported.	Yes	2

APPENDIX G. DATA ABSTRACTION OF PRIMARY STUDIES OBTAINED FROM GOOD QUALITY SYSTEMATIC REVIEWS RELATED TO PHARMACOTHERAPY

Author Year of systematic review	Time period and databases searched in systematic review	Eligibility criteria in systematic review	Study designs of eligible studies	Countries included in eligible studies	Sample size in eligible studies	Population in eligible studies	Interventions in eligible studies	Main results of eligible studies
Asenjo Lobos 2010[80]	Cochrane Schizophrenia Group's Trials Register: Inception–June 2007	RCTs, single- or double-blinded, comparing clozapine with other atypical antipsychotics for treatment of psychotic mental illness	No eligible RCTs	No eligible RCTs	No eligible RCTs	No eligible RCTs	No eligible RCTs	No eligible RCTs
Barbui 2009[82]	MEDLINE, EMBASE: January 1990–June 2008	Observational and case control; completed or attempted suicide; participants any sex and age with a diagnosis of MDD	No eligible RCTs	No eligible RCTs	No eligible RCTs	No eligible RCTs	No eligible RCTs	No eligible RCTs
Barbui 2008[81]	Cochrane Collaboration Depression, Anxiety and Neurosis Controlled Trials Register and the Cochrane Central Register of Controlled Trials: Inception-December 2006; MEDLINE: 1966-2006; EMBASE: 1974-2006	RCTs comparing paroxetine to placebo; participants were adults (≥18 years of age) of either sex with a diagnosis of major depression using any criteria	One RCT: DeRubeis 2005[23]	US	240	Adult civilians with moderate to severe major depressive disorder	Paroxetine vs. cognitive therapy vs. placebo	Suicide deaths: Paroxetine=1/120 (0.8%); Cognitive Therapy=0/60; Placebo=0/60
Cipriani 2005 (Fluoxetine)[83]	Cochrane Collaboration Depression, Anxiety, and Neurosis Controlled Trials Registers: Inception-2004; MEDLINE: 1966-2004; EMBASE: 1974-2004	RCTs; participants any sex and age with a primary diagnosis of depression	No eligible RCTs	No eligible RCTs	No eligible RCTs	No eligible RCTs	No eligible RCTs	No eligible RCTs
Cipriani 2005 (Lithium)[84]	Cochrane Collaboration Depression, Anxiety and Neurosis Controlled Trials Register, incorporating results of searches of MEDLINE (1966-June 2002); EMBASE: 1980-June 2002; CINAHL: 1982-March 2001; PsycLIT: 1974-June 2002; PSYNDEX: 1977-October 1999; LILACS: 1982-March 2001; CCRCT: 1999-2003	RCTs comparing lithium with placebo or all other compounds used in long-term (>3 months) treatment for mood disorders (unipolar depression, bipolar disorder, schizoaffective disorder, dysthymia, and rapid cycling, diagnosed according to Diagnostic and Statistical Manual of Mental Disorders [DSM] and International Classification of Diseases criteria)	No eligible RCTs	No eligible RCTs	No eligible RCTs	No eligible RCTs	No eligible RCTs	No eligible RCTs
Cipriani 2009[85]	Cochrane Collaboration Depression, Anxiety, and Neurosis Controlled Trials Registers: Inception-February 9, 2005	Prospective RCTs in any language comparing long-term treatment with lithium to any antidepressant	No eligible RCTs	No eligible RCTs	No eligible RCTs	No eligible RCTs	No eligible RCTs	No eligible RCTs
Dubicka 2010[87]	PsycINFO, MEDLINE, Cochrane databases: January 1980-March 2009	RCTs predominantly including adolescents aged 11-18 years with a DSM-IV defined episode of depression where CBT was combined with a newer generation antidepressant and compared with antidepressant treatment without CBT	No eligible RCTs	No eligible RCTs	No eligible RCTs	No eligible RCTs	No eligible RCTs	No eligible RCTs

---

Author Year of systematic review	Time period and databases searched in systematic review	Eligibility criteria in systematic review	Study designs of eligible studies	Countries included in eligible studies	Sample size in eligible studies	Population in eligible studies	Interventions in eligible studies	Main results of eligible studies
McDonagh 2010[92]	CCRCT: 1st Quarter 2010; CDSR: 4th Quarter 2009; MEDLINE: 1950-January week 4 2010; PsycINFO: 1806-February week 1 2010	RCTs, good quality systematic reviews, comparative observational studies; adults and adolescents with psychotic disorders; adults, children, and adolescents with major depressive disorder; adults with bipolar disorder; children and adolescents with disruptive behavior disorders; and older adults with dementia	No eligible RCTs	No eligible RCTs	No eligible RCTs	No eligible RCTs	No eligible RCTs	No eligible RCTs
National Collaborating Centre for Mental Health 2005[100]	MEDLINE, EMBASE, PsycINFO, Cochrane Library: Inception to September 2004	RCTs of depressed participants aged 5-18 treated with CBT, CBT+separate parenting sessions, interpersonal psychotherapy, psychoanalytic/psychodynamic child psychotherapy, self-modeling, relaxation, social skills training, family therapy, guided self-help, or control enhancement training; and that reported remission, symptom levels, functional status or discontinuation from treatment for any reason outcomes	No eligible RCTs	No eligible RCTs	No eligible RCTs	No eligible RCTs	No eligible RCTs	No eligible RCTs
Van Lieshout 2010[97]	MEDLINE: 1950-January week 2 2008; EMBASE: 1980-week 4 2008; PsycINFO: 1967-January week 2 2008; CINAHL: 1982-January week 2 2008; CCRCT, CDSR: 1800-2008	Published double-blind RCTs, placebo-controlled and active comparator trials (excluded crossover designs); included a mood stabilizer treatment group; adults aged 18-65 with bipolar disorder and acute major depression (excluded mixed states); Jadad scale score ≥3	One RCT: Calabrese 2005[28]	US	542	Adult civilians with acute bipolar depression	Mood stabilizer vs. placebo	Attempted suicides: Quetiapine 300 mg=1/172 (0.6%); Quetiapine 600 mg=1/170 (0.6%); Placebo=0/169
Williams 2009[98] & Williams 2009[99]	DARE, CDSR, MEDLINE, PsycINFO: 1998-May 2006	Patients aged 7-18 years with MDD or depression NOS; primary care setting, school-based clinics; English language only; excluded poor quality studies	Two RCTs: Emslie 2006[18] Wagner 2006[22]	US and Canada	206; 268	Child and adolescent civilians with a diagnosis of depression; Ages 6-17; Ages 7-17	SSRIs vs. placebo	No suicide deaths occurred in controlled trials of SSRIs

61

APPENDIX H. SUMMARY OF SYSTEMATIC REVIEW RESULTS RELATED TO PHARMACOTHERAPY FROM GAYNES ET AL., MANN ET AL., AND NICE REVIEWS[9-11]

	Gaynes 2004[9]	Mann 2005[10]	NICE 2011[11]
Overall conclusions	The poor generalizability of the studies makes the overall strength of evidence fair, at best, while the results are mixed. Although some trends suggest incremental benefit from several interventions, no consistent statistically significant effects have emerged for interventions for which more than one study has been done.	Interventions need more evidence of efficacy.	The evidence base for the pharmacological treatment for self-harm remains very limited. The clinical efficacy of these medications remains uncertain. The variations in the treatment lengths, follow-up period, and participants' psychiatric diagnosis in these trials made it more difficult to warrant conclusions about the clinical effects of these medications.
		Scope	
Search dates	1966–October 2002	1966–June 2005	Up to January 2011
Populations included	Population of interest was primary care patients with previously unidentified suicide risk. Included RCTs were conducted in high-risk groups as identified by a deliberate self-harm episode, diagnosis of borderline personality disorder, or admission to a psychiatric unit.	Not specified	Adults, children, and young people with previous self-harm behavior
Interventions included	Pharmacotherapy, psychotherapy, referral/follow-up	Pharmacotherapy, psychotherapy, referral/follow-up	Pharmacotherapy, psychotherapy, referral/follow-up
Suicide-related outcomes included	Suicide completions, suicide attempts	Completed and attempted suicide	Primary outcome was repetition of self-harm; also included suicide outcomes.
Settings/countries included	Primary or specialty care settings; no exclusions based on country.	Included settings not specified; no exclusions based on country.	No exclusions by country
Other exclusion criteria	Clinical trials targeting patients with chronic psychotic illnesses; studies without adequate comparison groups.	No additional exclusion criteria specified.	
		Main Results: Pharmacotherapy	
Antidepressants	Meta-analysis showed no statistically significant effects. No benefit for fluoxetine vs placebo in patients without major depression with 2 more suicide attempts.	Meta-analyses of RCTS have generally not detected benefit for suicide or suicide attempts in mood and other psychiatric disorders.	Insufficient evidence for suicide and self-harm
Antipsychotics	Flupenthixol significantly reduced the proportion of repeated deliberate self-harm for those with at least 2 previous suicide attempts compared with placebo. No benefit for low-dose vs. ultra low-dose fluphenazine in nonpsychotic patients with a previous suicide attempt.	Benefit for clozapine in people with schizophrenia spectrum disorders in 2 RCTs.	One RCT provides limited evidence of benefit of flupenthixol on self-harm repetition prevention compared to placebo, though no recommendation was made due to study limitations and potential harms. One RCT provides insufficient evidence of benefit of fluphenazine on reducing repeated self-harm or suicide.
Mood stabilizers		One RCT showed an antisuicidal effect of lithium in major mood disorders.	One RCT resulted in no significant differences between lithium and placebo on repetition of self-harm. Though 3 cases of suicide in the placebo arm were compared to the 0 cases in the lithium arm, study limitations precluded making recommendations.
Omega-3 fatty acid supplements			One RCT reported no significant differences for self-harm repetition.

APPENDIX I. DESCRIPTION OF PRIMARY OUTCOMES AND INTENT TO TREAT SUICIDAL SELF-DIRECTED VIOLENCE FOR PHARMACOTHERAPY STUDIES

Study, Year	Designed to treat suicide? (yes/no/unclear)	N	Outcome definition	Results
Berman 2007[29]	Unclear; suicide outcomes reported in results only.	362	Suicide Assessment methods NR	Suicides: None
Brent 2009[26]	Yes; the primary outcome was the occurrence of a suicidal adverse event.	334	Suicide-related symptoms assessed by the Beck Depression Inventory, Suicide Ideation Questionnaire-Jr., and Side Effects Form for Children and Adolescents.	Suicidal self-injury adverse events: No statistically significant treatment effects (rates NR)
Calabrese 2005[28]	Unclear; suicide outcomes reported in results only.	542	Suicide attempts, suicides: Assessment methods NR	Suicide attempts: 0.5% (1/180) vs 0.5% (1/181) vs. 0, P-value NR Suicides: None
DeRubeis 2005[23]	Unclear; suicide outcomes reported in results only.	240	Suicide Assessment methods NR	Suicide deaths: A=0.8% (1/120) vs B=0 vs C=0
Emslie 2006 (TADS)[19]	No; the objective of this article was to report adverse events, including suicide-related events, but suicide was not one of the pre-specified outcomes in the TADS study.	439	Suicide behavior assessed using Columbia-Classification Algorithm for Suicidal Assessment (C-CASA).	12 weeks Suicide deaths: None Suicide attempts: A=1.8% (2/109), B=0.9% (1/111), C=1.9% (2/107), D=0% (0/112), "rates are not significantly different" (P not reported) 36 weeks Suicide deaths: None Suicide attempts: A=6.4% (7/109), B=3.6% (4/111), C=3.7% (4/107), D=5.4% (6/112), P not reported
Emslie 2006[18]	No; post hoc analyses were conducted on the incidence of AEs related to suicidality.	206	Suicide Assessment methods NR	Suicide behavior: A=2% (2/104) vs B=0
Emslie 2009[20]	Yes; investigators assessed whether an adverse event was suggestive of self-harm; categorized as suicide attempt, suicidal ideation, self-injurious behavior (non-suicidal), accidental overdose, or other.	316	Suicide Assessment methods NR	Adverse events suggestive of self-harm, with a suicidal tendency: (A) 0 (B) 0.6% (1/157)
Goodyer 2008[27]	Yes; All acts of self-harm, including attempted suicide and non-suicidal self-cutting, and suicidal thoughts were asked about and recorded.	208	All acts of self-harm were asked about and recorded. Suicidality was rated based on suicidality items from the K-SADS-PL or the Suicidality/Self-Harm section of the K-SADS-L.	Suicide acts: Week 6: SSRI-only=9.2% (9/98) vs SSRI+CBT=5.1% (5/98) Week 12: SSRI-only=8.0% (8/100) vs SSRI+CBT=6.9% (7/101) Week 28: SSRI-only= 6.4% (6/94) vs SSRI+CBT= 7.1% (7/98) Time–treatment interaction: OR 1.002 (95% CI, 0.93 to 1.08) Pooled treatment effect: OR 0.995 (95% CI, 0.45 to 2.21)
Grunebaum 2011[24]	Yes; the primary aim of this study was to collect pilot data to explore if an SSRI antidepressant medication would be different from the NDRI, bupropion, for reducing suicidal behavior, ideation, and neuropsychological measures of impulsivity.	78	Suicidal events were assessed with the Columbia Suicide History Form (Oquendo 2003).	Suicide deaths: None

Study, Year	Designed to treat suicide? (yes/no/unclear)	N	Outcome definition	Results
Hallahan 2007[35]	Yes; measured suicidality with the Overt Aggression Scale.	49	Suicidality was measured using the Overt Aggression Scale.	No completed acts of suicide during the study period
Khan 2011[33]	Yes; a primary outcome measure was the Sheehan-Suicidality Tracking Scale.	80	Suicidal behaviors assessed using clinician-administered Sheehan-Suicidality Tracking Scale (S-STS).	Suicide deaths: None Suicide attempts: None
Lauterbach 2008[34 a]	Yes; primary outcome was a composite of attempted suicides and deaths by suicide.	167	Suicidal acts assessed by participant report.	Suicide deaths: A= 0/84 (0%) B= 3/83 (3.6%) Suicide attempts: A=7/84 (8.3%) B=7/83 (8.4%) Suicide attempt or death by suicide (primary endpoint): A=7 (8.3%) B=10 (12.0%) Incidence rate per patient-year: A=12.7% B=21.7% Adjusted HR: 0.52 (0.19 to 1.44); P=0.206 Death by suicide (post hoc secondary endpoint): A=0 (0%) B=3 (3.6%) Incidence rate per patient-year: A=0 B=6.5% P=0.049
Marcus 2008[30]	Unclear, suicide outcomes reported in results only	381	Suicide: Assessment methods NR	Suicides: None
Oquendo 2011[32]	Yes; The primary outcome measures were time to suicide completion, time to suicide attempt, and time to suicide event.	98	Suicide completion: self-inflicted death for which there was evidence of at least some intent to end one's life Suicide attempt: potentially self-injurious behavior carried out with at least some intent to end one's life	Suicide deaths: None Suicide attempts: A=12% (6/49) vs B=16% (8/49); P-value not reported Time to suicide attempt: Log-rank test showed no differences
Wagner 2006[22]	No; a post hoc analysis of suicide-related events was conducted.	268	Suicide Assessment methods NR	No suicides
Zisook 2011[25]	Unclear; primary outcome was suicidal ideation; methods do not specify suicidal behavior as an outcome.	665	Not reported	Suicide deaths: None Suicide attempts: A=0 vs B=0 vs C=2.3% (4/173), P=0.0162

[a] This study was excluded due to the country in which it was conducted; it is included in this table as a background article for comparison and discussion purposes.

APPENDIX J. DATA ABSTRACTION FOR PRIMARY STUDIES RELATED TO PHARMACOTHERAPY

Author, Year Country	Diagnosis	Interventions	Duration	N	Mean age, % female, race (variance)	Outcome definition	Results
Berman 2007[29] US	Adults with major depressive disorder with incomplete response to standard	(A) Adjunctive aripiprazole 11.8 mg/day (mean) (B) Adjunctive placebo Both added to ongoing standard antidepressants	6 weeks	362	Age (SD): A=46.5 (10.6), B=44.2 (10.9) Female: A=61.5%, B=64.2% Caucasian: A=87.4%, B=92.6% Black: A=8.2%, B=5.7%	Suicide Assessment methods NR	Suicides: None
Brent 2009[26] (TORDIA) US	SSRI-resistant depression in adolescents	Switch to another SSRI or venlafaxine: (A) With CBT (B) Without CBT	12 weeks	334	Mean age, years (SD): SSRI=16.0 (1.6), Venlafaxine=15.8 (1.5), No CBT=15.8 (1.6), CBT=16.0 (1.5) 70% Female 82% White	Suicide-related symptoms assessed by the Beck Depression Inventory, Suicide Ideation Questionnaire-Jr, and Side Effects Form for Children and Adolescents	Suicidal self-injury adverse events: No statistically significant treatment effects (rates NR)
Calabrese 2005[28] US	Adults with bipolar I or II depression	(A) Quetiapine 600 mg (B) Quetiapine 300 mg (C) Placebo	8 weeks	542	Age (SD): A=37.3 (11.4), B=36.6 (11.2), C=38.3 (11.1) Female: A=58.2%, B=54.1%, C=62.1% Caucasian: A=84.7%, B=82.0%, C=76.3% Black: A=10.6%, B=13.4%, C=15.4%	Suicide attempts, suicides: Assessment methods NR	Suicide attempts: 0.5% (1/180) vs 0.5% (1/181) vs 0, P-value NR Suicides: None
DeRubeis 2005[23] US	Adults with moderate to severe depression	(A) Paroxetine 10 mg to 50 mg (B) Placebo (C) Cognitive Therapy	8 weeks	240	Mean age (SD): 40 years (12) 59% Female 82% White	Suicide Assessment methods NR	Suicide deaths: A=0.8% (1/120) vs B=0 vs C=0
Emslie 2006 (TADS)[19] US	Adolescents with MDD	(A) Fluoxetine alone (B) CBT alone (C) Combination of fluoxetine and CBT (D) Placebo	36 weeks	439	Mean age (SD): 14.6 years (1.5) 54.4% Female 73.8% White 12.5% African American 8.9% Hispanic	Suicide behavior assessed using Columbia-Classification Algorithm for Suicidal Assessment (C-CASA)	12 weeks Suicide deaths: None Suicide attempts: A=1.8% (2/109), B=0.9% (1/111), C=1.9% (2/107), D=0% (0/112), "rates are not significantly different" (P not reported) 36 weeks Suicide deaths: None Suicide attempts: A=6.4% (7/109), B=3.6% (4/111), C=3.7% (4/107), D=5.4% (6/112), P not reported
Emslie 2006[18] US, Canada	Children and adolescents with MDD	(A) Paroxetine 10 mg (B) Placebo	8 weeks	206	Mean age (SD): 12.0 (2.97) 46.8% Female 79.3% White 20.7% Other race	Suicide Assessment methods NR	Suicide behavior: A=2% (2/104) vs B=0
Emslie 2009[20] US	Adolescent depression	(A) Escitalopram 10 to 20 mg (B) Placebo	8 weeks	316	Mean age (SD): A=14.7 (1.6) vs B=14.5 (1.5) % Female: A=59.4% vs B=58.6% White: A=72.9% vs B=78.3%	Suicide Assessment methods NR	Adverse events suggestive of self-harm, with a suicidal tendency: (A) 0 (B) 0.6% (1/157)

Author, Year Country	Diagnosis	Interventions	Duration	N	Mean age, % female, race (variance)	Outcome definition	Results
Goodyer 2008 (ADAPT)[27] UK	Adolescents with MDD	(A) SSRI alone (fluoxetine treatment of choice) (B) SSRI plus CBT	28 weeks	208	Mean age (SD): 14.0 years (1.5) 74% Female 97% were of white European origin	All acts of self-harm were asked about and recorded. Suicidality was rated based on suicidality items from the K-SADS-PL or the Suicidality/Self-Harm section of the K-SADS-L	Suicide acts: Week 6: SSRI-only=9.2% (9/98) vs SSRI+CBT=5.1% (5/98) Week 12: SSRI-only=8.0% (8/100) vs SSRI+CBT=6.9% (7/101) Week 28: SSRI-only= 6.4% (6/94) vs SSRI+CBT= 7.1% (7/98) Time-treatment interaction: OR 1.002 (95% CI, 0.93 to 1.08) Pooled treatment effect: OR 0.995 (95% CI, 0.45 to 2.21)
Grunebaum 2011[24] US	Adults with MDD with a suicide attempt history or current suicidal ideation	(A) Bupropion (B) Paroxetine	Acute=8 weeks Continuation=16 weeks	78	Mean age, years (SD): A=37.9 (11.9) vs B=35.2 (12.8) % Female: A=55.3% vs B=58.3% White: A=68.4% vs B=72.2%	Suicidal events were assessed with the Columbia Suicide History Form (Oquendo 2003)	Suicide deaths: None
Hallahan 2007[35] Ireland	Adults who presented acutely with self-harm	(A) Eicosapentaenoic acid 1.2 mg plus docosahexaenoic acid 0.9 mg (B) Placebo	12 weeks	49	Age, mean: A=30.5 vs B=30.7 65% Female Race NR	Suicidality was measured using the Overt Aggression Scale	No completed acts of suicide during the study period
Khan 2011[33] US	Severely ill depressed adults	(A) Citalopram 20 mg plus lithium 300 mg (B) Citalopram 20 mg plus placebo	4 weeks	80	Age, mean: A=45.0 vs B=38.5 % Female: A=47.5% vs B=62.5% % Caucasian: A=72.5% vs B=62.5%	Suicidal behaviors assessed using clinician-administered Sheehan-Suicidality Tracking Scale (S-STS)	Suicide deaths: None Suicide attempts: None
Lauterbach 2008[34] Germany[a]	Adults with a suicide attempt within 3 months in the context of a depressive spectrum disorder (76% major depressive disorder, 19% adjustment disorder, 5% other (e.g., dysthymia)	(A) Lithium (effective blood level considered 0.6-0.8 mmol/l (B) Placebo	1 year	167	A vs B: Mean age (SD): 39.6 (3.9) vs 39.3 (13.0) 61.9% vs 53.0% female Race NR	Attempted suicides and deaths by suicide (composite): Suicidal acts assessed by participant report.	Suicide deaths: A=0/84 (0%) B=3/83 (3.6%) Suicide attempts: A=7/84 (8.3%) B=7/83 (8.4%) *Suicide attempt or death by suicide (primary endpoint):* A=7 (8.3%) B=10 (12.0%) Incidence rate per patient-year: A=12.7% B=21.7% Adjusted HR: 0.52 (0.19 to 1.44); P=0.206 *Death by suicide (post hoc secondary endpoint):* A=0 (0%) B=3 (3.6%) Incidence rate per patient-year: A=0 B=6.5% P=0.049

Author, Year Country	Diagnosis	Interventions	Duration	N	Mean age, % female, race (variance)	Outcome definition	Results
Marcus 2008[30] US	Adults with major depressive disorder with incomplete response to standard	(A) Adjunctive aripiprazole 11.0 mg/day (mean) (B) Adjunctive placebo Both added to ongoing standard antidepressants	6 weeks	381	Age (SD): A=44.6 (11.0), B=44.4 (10.7) Female: A=66.0%, B=67.4% Caucasian: A=89.0%, B=88.9% Black: A=7.3%, B=7.4%	Suicide: Assessment methods NR	Suicides: None
Oquendo 2011[32] US	Adults with bipolar disorder, in a depressive or mixed episode, with ≥ 1 past suicide attempt	(A) Lithium 0.6–1.0 mEq/dl (B) Valproate 45–125 μg/ml Open-label adjunctive treatment provided as needed, based on algorithm	2.5 years	98	Age, mean (SD): A=33 (11) vs B=34 (10) % Female: A=76% vs B=69% % White: A=67% vs B=64%	Suicide completion: self-inflicted death for which there was evidence of at least some intent to end one's life Suicide attempt: potentially self-injurious behavior carried out with at least some intent to end one's life	Suicide deaths: None Suicide attempts: A=12% (6/49) vs B=16% (8/49); P-value not reported Time to suicide attempt: Log-rank test showed no differences
Wagner 2006[22] US	Children with MDD	(A) Escitalopram 10-20 mg (B) Placebo	8 weeks	268	Mean age (SD): A=12.2 (3.9) vs B=12.4 (3.0) % female: A=51.9% vs B=51.9% White: A=71.0% vs B=71.4% Black: A=14.5% vs B=12.8% Asian: A=0.8% vs B=1.5% Other: A=13.7% vs B=14.3%	Suicide Assessment methods NR	No suicides
Zisook 2011[25] US	Adults with either recurrent or chronic MDD	(A) Escitalopram plus placebo (B) Escitalopram plus bupropion SR (C) Venlafaxine XR plus mirtazapine	7 months	665	Mean age (SD): 42.7 years (13.0) 68% Female 67% White 27.1% Black 15.2% Hispanic 5.9% Other	Not reported	Suicide deaths: None Suicide attempts: A=0 vs B=0 vs C=2.3% (4/173), P=0.0162

[a] This study was excluded due to the country in which it was conducted; it is included in this table as a background article for comparison and discussion purposes only.

APPENDIX K. RISK OF BIAS RATINGS FOR PRIMARY STUDIES RELATED TO PHARMACOTHERAPY

Author Year	Sequence generation — Describe method	Sequence generation — Was it adequate? Yes/No/Unclear	Allocation concealment — Describe method	Allocation concealment — Was it adequate? Yes/No/Unclear	Blinding of participants, personnel, and outcome assessors — Describe all measures used, if any, to blind study participants and personnel from knowledge of which intervention participant received. Provide any information relating to whether intended blinding was effective.	Blinding — Was knowledge of allocated intervention adequately prevented during study? Yes/No/Unclear	Incomplete outcome data — Describe completeness of outcome data for each main outcome, including attrition and exclusions from analysis. State whether attrition and exclusions were reported, numbers in each intervention group (compared with total randomized participants), reasons for attrition/exclusions where reported and any re-inclusions in analyses performed by review authors.	Incomplete outcome data — Were incomplete outcome data adequately addressed? Yes/No/Unclear	Selective outcome reporting — State how possibility of selective outcome reporting was examined by review authors and what was found.	Selective outcome reporting — Are reports of study free of suggestion of selective outcome reporting? Yes/No/Unclear	Other sources of bias — State any important concerns about bias not addressed in other domains in tool. If particular questions/entries were pre-specified in review's protocol, responses should be provided for each question/entry.	Other sources of bias — Was study apparently free of other problems that could put it at high risk of bias? Yes/No/Unclear	OVERALL risk of bias for study as a whole — Low/Unclear/High
Berman 2007[29]	Method not described	Unclear	Method not described	Unclear	Described as double-blind, but no information about appearance or whether outcome assessors were blinded.	Unclear	For safety analyses, Intention-to-treat (ITT) using Last Observation Carried Forward (LOCF) of all who received double-blind treatment (99%); overall attrition=10%; placebo=9.1% vs aripiprazole=12.1%.	Yes	Protocol available on clinicaltrials. gov, but minimal detail about outcomes provided.	Unclear	No important concerns.	Yes	Unclear
Brent 2009[28]	"Subjects were randomly assigned to one of four conditions in a 2-by-2 factorial design.... Subjects were assigned to treatment using a variation of Efron's biased coin toss, balancing both across and within sites."	Yes	No information provided	Unclear	"The intent was for study participants, clinicians, and independent evaluators to be blinded to medication treatment assignment, and for independent evaluators to be blinded to CBT assignment." Use of triple-dummy. "The pharmacotherapists' accuracy in guessing medication assignment was less accurate than chance (44.2%; z=4.57; P=.03), whereas the independent evaluators guessed CBT assignment at a rate slightly higher than chance (58.3%; z=5.14; P=.02). In 64 cases, the blinding of the independent evaluator was compromised, most commonly because of participant disclosure of receiving CBT." Study was designed to compare the relative efficacy of well-matched treatment alternatives and, therefore, even though patients may have been aware of the type of treatment they were receiving, all treatments were likely perceived as effective treatment methods.	Participants=yes to meds, no for CBT Personnel=yes for meds, no for CBT Assessors=unclear	Missing data, attritions, and exclusions adequately reported. Rates of treatment completion were reported with respect to primary outcomes. ITT using LOCF; attrition: overall=31%, venlafaxine alone=27%, venlafaxine with CBT=36%, SSRI alone=29%, SSRI with CBT=30%.	Yes	Protocol available on clinicaltrials.gov, but planned outcomes were not provided, and all expected suicide-related outcomes were reported.	Yes	Midway through the study, the paroxetine treatment option in the SSRI group was changed to citalopram due to safety concerns about paroxetine. Also, midway through the study the method for monitoring, self-harm was changed from spontaneous report to proactive assessment. No information is provided re: possible nested (e.g., therapist) effects.	Unclear	Unclear

Author Year	Sequence generation		Allocation concealment		Blinding of participants, personnel, and outcome assessors		Incomplete outcome data		Selective outcome reporting		Other sources of bias		OVERALL risk of bias for study as a whole
	Describe method	Was it adequate? Yes/No/ Unclear	Describe method	Was it adequate? Yes/No/ Unclear	Describe all measures used, if any, to blind study participants and personnel from knowledge of which intervention participant received. Provide any information relating to whether intended blinding was effective.	Was knowledge of allocated intervention adequately prevented during study? Yes/No/ Unclear	Describe completeness of outcome data for each main outcome, including attrition and exclusions from analysis. State whether attrition and exclusions were reported, numbers in each intervention group (compared with total randomized participants), reasons for attrition/exclusions where reported and any re-inclusions in analyses performed by review authors.	Were incomplete outcome data adequately addressed? Yes/No/ Unclear	State how possibility of selective outcome reporting was examined by review authors and what was found.	Are reports of study free of suggestion of selective outcome reporting? Yes/No/ Unclear	State any important concerns about bias not addressed in other domains in tool. If particular questions/ entries were pre-specified in review's protocol, responses should be provided for each question/ entry.	Was study apparently free of other problems that could put it at high risk of bias? Yes/No/ Unclear	Low/Unclear/ High
Calabrese 2005[28]	Insufficient information.	Unclear	Random assignment was achieved in a non-center-specific manner with an interactive voice-response central randomization service.	Yes	Described as double-blind and use of identically-appearing tablets is considered sufficient for blindings of study personnel and patient, but no information about blinding of outcome assessor. Also noted that "moderate rates of sedation or somnolence were observed in both quetiapine groups, which might have compromised the integrity of the double-blind design," but lower likelihood that suicide assessment was influenced by inadequate blinding.	Unclear	No missing outcome data.	Yes	No omissions of any expected suicide-related outcomes.	Yes	The study appears to be free of other sources of bias.	Yes	Low
DeRubeis 2005[23]	Not described.	Unclear	Not described.	Unclear	Outcome assessors were blinded to all treatment conditions. Patients and pharmacotherapists were blinded to pharmacotherapy during first 8 weeks; patients and therapists were not blinded to cognitive therapy assignment.	Outcome assessors= yes. Patients/ therapists in pharmacotherapy groups= unclear. Patients/ therapists in cognitive therapy group=no.	ITT with LOCF; attrition was reasonable (13% in first 8 weeks; 5% in second 8 weeks); numbers and reasons were balanced across groups.	Yes	Protocol not available.	Unclear	None noted.	Yes	Unclear
Emslie 2006 (TADS)[19]	Computerized randomization.	Yes	No information provided.	Unclear	"Participants and all study staff remained masked in the pills-only conditions (FLX and PBO) until the end of stage I (week 12). Patients and treatment providers in COMB and CBT were aware of treatment assignment." "The primary dependent measures rated blindly by an independent evaluator are the Children's Depression Rating Scale and, for responder analysis, a dichotomized Clinical Global Impressions-Improvement score." Notably, the study was designed to compare the relative efficacy of well-matched treatment alternatives and, therefore, even though patients may have been aware of the type of treatment they were receiving, all treatments were likely perceived as effective treatment methods.	Unclear	Well-described ITT analysis and pre-treatment group comparisons included in article. No missing outcome data reported. Attritions and exclusions adequately documented, and subject flowchart included in article.	Yes	No omissions of any expected suicide-related outcomes.	Yes	The study appears to be free of other sources of bias. Well-described statistical accounting for potential nested data effects through the use of random effects modeling.	Yes	Unclear

Author Year	Sequence generation — Describe method	Was it adequate? Yes/No/Unclear	Allocation concealment — Describe method	Was it adequate? Yes/No/Unclear	Blinding of participants, personnel, and outcome assessors — Describe all measures used, if any, to blind study participants and personnel from knowledge of which intervention participant received. Provide any information relating to whether intended blinding was effective.	Was knowledge of allocated intervention adequately prevented during study? Yes/No/Unclear	Incomplete outcome data — Describe completeness of outcome data for each main outcome, including attrition and exclusions from analysis. State whether attrition and exclusions were reported, numbers in each intervention group (compared with total randomized participants), reasons for attrition/exclusions where reported and any re-inclusions in analyses performed by review authors.	Were incomplete outcome data adequately addressed? Yes/No/Unclear	Selective outcome reporting — State how possibility of selective outcome reporting was examined by review authors and what was found.	Are reports of study free of suggestion of selective outcome reporting? Yes/No/Unclear	Other sources of bias — State any important concerns about bias not addressed in other domains in tool. If particular questions/entries were pre-specified in review's protocol, responses should be provided for each question/entry.	Was study apparently free of other problems that could put it at high risk of bias? Yes/No/Unclear	OVERALL risk of bias for study as a whole Low/Unclear/High
Emslie 2006[18]	Computer generated.	Yes	No information provided.	Unclear	Described as double-blind, but no details provided about appearance of treatments or blinding of outcome assessors.	Unclear	ITT using LOCF; overall attrition=18%, numbers and reasons balanced across groups.	Yes	Protocol available on clinicaltrials.gov. Primary outcome was consistent and reported; but only one secondary outcome was listed in protocol and many others were reported in publication.	Unclear	No concerns.	Yes	Unclear
Emslie 2009[20]	No information provided.	Unclear	No information provided.	Unclear	Described as double-blind, but no explicit statement about who was blinded. No information about appearance of tablets.	Unclear	ITT using LOCF; safety analyses included all patients who received ≥ 1 dose of study medication (99%); efficacy analyses included all patients in safety analyses who had ≥ 1 post-baseline assessment. Attrition: overall=18% in 8-week study; placebo=16%, escitalopram=20%.	Yes	Protocol available on clinicaltrials.gov, and primary and secondary outcomes match, and were reported.	Yes	Free of other sources of bias.	Yes	Unclear
Goodyer 2008[27]	Stochastic minimization used to ensure balance (so probably computer-generated).	Unclear	Central allocation, controlled by independent center.	Yes	Participants and treating clinicians: not blinded. Outcome assessment done by independent evaluators blind to treatment assignment. Participants, parents and treating clinicians instructed not to disclose treatment assignments. Adequacy of blinding tested by asking evaluators to guess treatment assignment, but results of testing NR.	Participants and treating clinicians=no. Outcome assessors= unclear.	ITT; overall attrition=15%, numbers balanced between groups. Reasons were not separated by group, but predictors of missing data were included as covariates in the statistical analyses.	Yes	Protocol not available.	Unclear	None noted.	Yes	Unclear
Grunebaum 2011[24]	Computer-generated.	Yes	Sequence generated by a pharmacist separate from research team.	Unclear (probably yes)	Patients, psychiatrists and assessors were blinded to treatment. Pills were identically over-encapsulated so patients were blinded. After 8 weeks, the 16-week continuation phase remained blinded if patient had a satisfactory response; otherwise they were switched to open treatment.	Yes for acute phase; no for those switched to open-label treatment in continuation phase.	Modified ITT, excluded 5% (3/78 due to ineligibility discovered after randomization, 1/78 lost to follow-up after randomization visit); high attrition (68%), but balanced across groups in numbers and reasons.	Unclear	Protocol not available.	Unclear	Only 27% completed 24 weeks on assigned medication.	Yes	Unclear

70

Author Year	Sequence generation		Allocation concealment		Blinding of participants, personnel, and outcome assessors		Incomplete outcome data		Selective outcome reporting		Other sources of bias		OVERALL risk of bias for study as a whole
	Describe method	Was it adequate? Yes/No/Unclear	Describe method	Was it adequate? Yes/No/Unclear	Describe all measures used, if any, to blind study participants and personnel from knowledge of which intervention participant received. Provide any information relating to whether intended blinding was effective.	Was knowledge of allocated intervention adequately prevented during study? Yes/No/Unclear	Describe completeness of outcome data for each main outcome, including attrition and exclusions from analysis. State whether attrition and exclusions were reported, numbers in each intervention group (compared with total randomized participants), reasons for attrition/exclusions where reported and any re-inclusions in analyses performed by review authors.	Were incomplete outcome data adequately addressed? Yes/No/Unclear	State how possibility of selective outcome reporting was examined by review authors and what was found.	Are reports of study free of suggestion of selective outcome reporting? Yes/No/Unclear	State any important concerns about bias not addressed in other domains in tool. If particular questions/entries were pre-specified in review's protocol, responses should be provided for each question/entry.	Was study apparently free of other problems that could put it at high risk of bias? Yes/No/Unclear	Low/Unclear/High
Hallahan 2007[35]	Computer-generated list.	Yes	Dispensed by an independent colleague; code only revealed once data collection was complete.	Yes	Identical capsules, ensured equality of "fishy breath".	Yes	ITT using LOCF; attrition: overall=20%, placebo=26%, omega-3 fatty acid=14%.	Yes	Protocol not available. All expected suicide-related outcomes were reported.	Yes	Free of other sources of bias.	Yes	Low
Khan 2011[33]	Computer program.	Yes	Central allocation, controlled by independent pharmacist.	Yes	Double-blind: Patients and key study personnel. Blinding ensured by use of "closely matching" placebo and matching prescription bottles. Not explicitly stated that clinician was blinded.	Unclear for all	ITT using LOCF; Attrition=20%; numbers and reasons balanced across groups	Yes	Protocol not available.	Unclear	None noted.	Yes	Low
Lauterbach 2008[34] a	Computerized randomization sequence.	Yes	Not described.	Unclear	Double-blinded assessment was conducted, although in some cases this procedure could not be maintained because of emergencies in relation to suicidal acts or insufficient drug compliance.	No	56/84 (67%) lithium and 59/83 (71%) placebo lost to follow-up by 12 months. Did ITT analysis. Recruitment was only 36% of that estimated required for adequate power 167/468. 7 patients in treatment group and 10 in control group with suicide or suicide attempts were counted as lost to follow-up.	No; although ITT analysis was done, loss to follow-up was very high.	Primary outcome was a composite of suicide and suicide attempts; suicidal acts were determined by self-report only. Did a post hoc analysis of deaths by suicides (showing 3 in placebo group vs 0 in lithium group) and this finding is highlighted even though there was no significant difference found on the primary outcome.	No	Differences between groups at baseline on important prognostic factors: more patients in the lithium group had personality disorders (53% vs 31%; P=0.12); more in the lithium group had multiple prior suicide attempts (57% vs 31%; P=0.001); and patients in the lithium group had higher scores on the suicide intent scale at their index attempt (P=0.046).	No	High

Author Year	Sequence generation		Allocation concealment		Blinding of participants, personnel, and outcome assessors		Incomplete outcome data		Selective outcome reporting		Other sources of bias		OVERALL risk of bias for study as a whole
	Describe method	Was it adequate? Yes/No/Unclear	Describe method	Was it adequate? Yes/No/Unclear	Describe all measures used, if any, to blind study participants and personnel from knowledge of which intervention participant received. Provide any information relating to whether intended blinding was effective.	Was knowledge of allocated intervention adequately prevented during study? Yes/No/Unclear	Describe completeness of outcome data for each main outcome, including attrition and exclusions from analysis. State whether attrition and exclusions were reported, numbers in each intervention group (compared with total randomized participants), reasons for attrition/exclusions where reported and any re-inclusions in analyses performed by review authors.	Were incomplete outcome data adequately addressed? Yes/No/Unclear	State how possibility of selective outcome reporting was examined by review authors and what was found.	Are reports of study free of suggestion of selective outcome reporting? Yes/No/Unclear	State any important concerns about bias not addressed in other domains in tool. If particular questions/ entries were pre-specified in review's protocol, responses should be provided for each question/ entry.	Was study apparently free of other problems that could put it at high risk of bias? Yes/No/Unclear	Low/Unclear/High
Marcus 2008[30]	Method not described.	Unclear	Method not described.	Unclear	Described as double-blind, but no information about appearance or whether outcome assessors were blinded.	Unclear	For safety analyses, ITT using LOCF of all who received double-blind treatment (100%); overall attrition=15%; placebo=14.7% vs aripiprazole=15.2%.	Yes	No protocol available.	Unclear	No important concerns.	Yes	Unclear
Oquendo 2011[32]	Not described.	Unclear	Not described.	Unclear	"Patients, study psychiatrists, and assessors were blind to treatment assignment." Double-dummy approach used. Lithium levels monitored by nontreating physician.	Yes	46/48 lithium and 48/49 valpoate included in analysis. Used ITT analysis, but high loss to follow-up and those lost to follow-up had more previous psychiatric hospitalizations and were more likely to report a history of childhood abuse.	Unclear	Unclear if study protocol is available. No clinicaltrials.gov number provided, but reported all expected outcomes.	Unclear	1) 6 patients were eligible but not randomzed for not enrolling notrepote 2) Power-analysis enrollment target not met. "However, the power analysis was based on an attempt rate much lower than that observed in this study."	Unclear	Unclear
Wagner 2006[22]	Computer-generated randomization schedule.	Yes	No information provided.	Unclear	Described as double-blind and use of identically-appearing tablets. No information about blinding of outcome assessor.	Participants/personnel: yes. Outcome assessor: unclear.	ITT using LOCF; attrition: overall=19%; numbers and reasons balanced across groups.	Yes	Protocol not available.	Unclear	No other concerns.	Yes	Unclear
Zisook 2011[25]	Web-based randomization system (reference is from STAR*D).	Yes	Not described.	Unclear	Participants: only blind to second medication. Study personnel: not blinded.	Participants: no to first medication, yes to second medication. Study personnel: no.	ITT; attrition: acute phase=23%, continuation phase=12%; reasons for attrition not reported.	Unclear	Protocol available at clinicaltrials.gov, but explicit identification of specific scales planned to measure primary and secondary outcomes was lacking.	Unclear	2 of 4 suicide attempts occurred during the continuation phase; it is possible those who did not continue differed from those who did.	Unclear	Unclear

a This study was excluded due to the country in which it was conducted; it is included in this table as a background article for comparison and discussion purposes only.

APPENDIX L. STRENGTH OF EVIDENCE RATINGS FOR PRIMARY STUDIES RELATED TO PHARMACOTHERAPY[a]

Table 1: Antidepressants vs placebo

Number of studies; # of subjects	Domains pertaining to strength of evidence				Magnitude of effect	Strength of evidence
	Risk of bias (Design/ Risk of bias)	Consistency	Directness	Precision	Magnitude of effect	High, Moderate, Low, Insufficient
Escitalopram versus placebo (Emslie 2009, Wagner 2006)[20, 22]						
Suicide deaths (Wagner 2006)[22]						
1; 268	Medium (RCT/Unclear)	N/A	Indirect	Imprecise	No events	Insufficient
Adverse events suggestive of self-harm, with a suicidal tendency (Emslie 2009)[20]						
1; 316	Medium (RCT/Unclear)	N/A	Indirect	Imprecise	0 vs 0.6% (1/157)	Low
Fluoxetine versus placebo (TADS)[19, 21, 124, 125]						
Suicide deaths at 36 weeks						
1; 221	Low (RCT/Low)	N/A	Indirect	Imprecise	No events	Insufficient
Suicide attempts at 36 weeks						
1; 221	Low (RCT/Low)	N/A	Indirect	Imprecise	6.4% (7/109) vs 5.4% (6/112), *P* not reported	Low
Paroxetine versus placebo (DeRubeis 2005, Emslie 2006)[18, 23]						
Suicide deaths (DeRubeis 2005)[23]						
1; 180	Low (RCT/Low)	N/A	Indirect	Imprecise	0.8% (1/120) vs 0	Low
Suicide behavior (Emslie 2006)[18]						
1; 206	Low (RCT/Low)	N/A	Indirect	Imprecise	2% (2/104) vs 0	Low

Table 2: Antidepressants vs antidepressants

Number of studies; # of subjects	Domains pertaining to strength of evidence				Magnitude of effect	Strength of evidence
	Risk of bias (Design/ Risk of bias)	Consistency	Directness	Precision	Magnitude of effect	High, Moderate, Low, Insufficient
Escitalopram plus placebo vs escitalopram plus bupropion SR vs venlafaxine XR plus mirtazapine (Zisook 2011)[25]						
Suicide deaths						
1; 665	Medium (RCT/Unclear)	N/A	Indirect	Imprecise	No events	Insufficient
Suicide attempts						
1; 665	Medium (RCT/Unclear)	N/A	Indirect	Imprecise	0 vs 0 vs 2.3%, *P*=0.0162	Low
Bupropion vs paroxetine (Grunebaum 2011)[24]						
Suicide deaths						
1; 78	Medium (RCT/Unclear)	N/A	Indirect	Imprecise	No events	Insufficient

Table 3: Antidepressants alone vs antidepressants plus Cognitive Behavioral Therapy (CBT)

Number of studies; # of subjects	Domains pertaining to strength of evidence				Magnitude of effect	Strength of evidence
	Risk of bias (Design/ Risk of bias)	Consistency	Directness	Precision	Magnitude of effect	High, Moderate, Low, Insufficient
Fluoxetine alone vs fluoxetine plus CBT (TADS)[19, 21, 124, 125]						
Suicide deaths at 36 weeks						
1; 216	Medium (RCT/Unclear)	N/A	Indirect	Imprecise	No events	Insufficient
Suicide attempts at 36 weeks						
1; 216	Medium (RCT/Unclear)	N/A	Indirect	Imprecise	6.4% vs 3.7%, *P* not reported	Low
Switch to another SSRI or venlafaxine, with or without CBT (TORDIA)[26, 126]						
Suicidal self-injury adverse events at 12 weeks						
1; 334	Medium (RCT/Unclear)	N/A	Indirect	Imprecise	No statistically significant treatment effects (rates NR)	Low
SSRI alone (fluoxetine treatment of choice) vs SSRI plus CBT (ADAPT)[27]						
Suicide acts at 28 weeks						
1; 208	Medium (RCT/Unclear)	N/A	Indirect	Imprecise	6.4% vs 7.1%	Low

Table 4: Antidepressants versus Cognitive Behavioral Therapy (CBT)

Number of studies; # of subjects	Domains pertaining to strength of evidence				Magnitude of effect	Strength of evidence
	Risk of bias (Design/ Risk of bias)	Consistency	Directness	Precision	Magnitude of effect	High, Moderate, Low, Insufficient
Antidepressants versus CBT (DeRubeis 2005)[23]						
Suicide deaths						
1; 180	Medium (RCT/Unclear)	N/A	Indirect	Imprecise	0.8% vs 0	Low

Table 5: Atypical Antipsychotics

Number of studies; # of subjects	Domains pertaining to strength of evidence				Magnitude of effect	Strength of evidence
	Risk of bias (Design/ Risk of bias)	Consistency	Directness	Precision	Magnitude of effect	High, Moderate, Low, Insufficient
Quetiapine (Calabrese 2005)[28]						
Suicide attempts						
1; 542	Low (RCT/Low)	N/A	Indirect	Imprecise	0.5% (1/180) vs 0.5% (1/181) vs 0, P-value NR	Low
Suicides						
1; 542	Low (RCT/Low)	N/A	Indirect	Imprecise	No events	Low
Aripiprazole (Berman 2007, Marcus 2008)[29, 30]						
Suicides						
2; 743	Medium (RCT/Unclear)	Consistent	Indirect	Imprecise	No events	Low
Clozapine (Glick 2004 & Meltzer 2003 as cited in Mann 2005)[10]						
Unclear outcome in Mann 2005[10]						
2; not reported	Medium (RCT/Unclear due to lack of report)	Consistent	Indirect	N/A	Not reported	Insufficient to Low

Table 6: Mood stabilizers

Number of studies; # of subjects	Domains pertaining to strength of evidence				Magnitude of effect	Strength of evidence
	Risk of bias (Design/ Risk of bias)	Consistency	Directness	Precision	Magnitude of effect	High, Moderate, Low, Insufficient
Lithium versus valproate (Oquendo 2011)[32]						
Suicide deaths						
1; 98	Medium (RCT/Unclear)	N/A	Indirect	Imprecise	No events	Insufficient
Suicide attempts						
1; 98	Medium (RCT/Unclear)	N/A	Indirect	Imprecise	12% (6/49) vs 16% (8/49)	Low
Time to suicide attempt						
1; 98	Medium (RCT/Unclear)	N/A	Indirect	Imprecise	Log-rank test showed no differences	Low
Citalopram plus lithium versus citalopram plus placebo (Khan 2011)[33]						
Suicide deaths						
1; 80	Low (RCT/Low)	N/A	Indirect	Imprecise	No events	Insufficient
Suicide attempts						
1; 98	Low (RCT/Low)	N/A	Indirect	Imprecise	No events	Insufficient

Lithium versus placebo (Lauterbach 2008)[34]						
Suicide deaths						
1; 167	High (RCT/High)	N/A	Indirect	Imprecise	0% (0/84) 3.6% (3/83) Incidence rate per patient-year: 0% vs 6.5% P=0.049	Insufficient
Suicide attempts						
1; 167	High (RCT/High)	N/A	Indirect	Imprecise	8.3% (7/84) 8.4% (7/83) Not significant	Insufficient
Composite of suicide attempt/suicide death						
1; 167	High (RCT/High)	N/A	Indirect	Imprecise	Adjusted HR: 0.52 (0.19 to 1.44); P=0.206	Insufficient
Lithium (Theis-Flechtner 1996 as cited in Mann 2005)[10]						
Unclear outcome in Mann 2005						
1; not reported	Medium (RCT/ Unclear due to lack of report)	N/A	Indirect	N/A	Not reported	Insufficient to Low

Table 7: Omega-3 fatty acid supplementation vs placebo (Hallahan 2007)[35]

	Domains pertaining to strength of evidence				Magnitude of effect	Strength of evidence
Number of studies; # of subjects	**Risk of bias (Design/ Risk of bias)**	**Consistency**	**Directness**	**Precision**	**Magnitude of effect**	**High, Moderate, Low, Insufficient**
Suicide deaths						
1; 49	Low (RCT/Low)	N/A	Indirect	Imprecise	No events	Insufficient

[a] This review did not evaluate any outcomes other than suicidal self-directed violence and, therefore, no additional data on potential harms and side effects was investigated. Potential harms and side effects should always be considered when evaluating the strength of evidence and considering adoption of an intervention or referral/follow-up service.

APPENDIX M. QUALITY RATING OF SYSTEMATIC REVIEWS RELATED TO PSYCHOTHERAPY USING OXMAN AND GUYATT[15] CRITERIA

Author Year of systematic review	Search methods reported	Comprehensive search	Inclusion criteria reported	Selection bias avoided	Validity criteria reported	Validity assessed appropriately	Methods used to combine studies reported	Findings combined appropriately	Conclusions supported by data	Overall scientific quality (higher score is better)
Abbass 2009[102]	Yes	Yes	Yes	Yes	Yes	Yes	Yes	Yes	Yes	7
Binks 2011[104]	Yes	Yes	Yes	Yes	Yes	Yes	Yes	Yes	Yes	7
Corcoran 2011[105]	Yes	Yes	Yes	Yes	Yes	Can't tell; reported that 6 studies did not meet the quality criteria, but did not specify which studies, which criteria, and did not appear to do any type of sensitivity analysis.	Yes	Yes	Yes	5
Craig 2009[86]	No; no mention of search terms.	No; no supplemental sources.	Yes	No; detailed results of study selection not reported, no reasons for exclusions described.	No	Can't tell; within GRADE evaluation of quality of evidence, deducted points for internal validity limitations; but, unclear as to the scope of the internal validity domains assessed.	Yes	Yes	Yes	3
Dieterich 2010[106]	Yes	Yes; only searched one database, though this database combines multiple other databases.	Yes	Yes	Yes	Yes	Yes	Yes	Yes	7
Dubicka 2010[87]	Yes	Yes	Yes	Yes; study flow diagram provided reasons for exclusion.	Yes	Yes; reported results of validity assessment; none were poor, not necessarily a need to control for variation in synthesis.	Yes	Yes	Yes	7
Hazell 2011[89]	Partially; no mention of search terms.	No; no supplemental sources.	Yes	Can't tell; numbers and reasons for exclusions not reported	No	Yes, validity assessment included in GRADE strength of evidence ratings	Yes; used GRADE approach to rate strength of evidence	Yes	Yes	5
Innamorati 2011[90]	Yes	No; no supplemental sources.	No; no information on PICOTS.	Can't tell; only reported number of included studies.	No; none described; only use of Shekelle 1999[123] scheme for classifying study design and strength of recommendation, but no quality assessment	No	Yes; used Shekelle 1999[123] scheme for classifying study design and strength of recom-mendation	Yes	Yes	3

77

Author Year of systematic review	Search methods reported	Comprehensive search	Inclusion criteria reported	Selection bias avoided	Validity criteria reported	Validity assessed appropriately	Methods used to combine studies reported	Findings combined appropriately	Conclusions supported by data	Overall scientific quality (higher score is better)
Irving 2010[107]	Yes	Yes	Yes	Yes	Yes	Yes	Yes	Yes	Yes	7
Kavanagh 2009[108]	Partially; date of most recent searches not reported.	Yes	Yes	Yes	Yes	Yes	Yes	Yes	Yes	7
Lapierre 2011[109]	Yes	Yes	Yes	Can't tell; detailed results of study selection not reported, no reasons for exclusion described.	Yes	No; reported validity assessment, but did not do any type of analysis with it.	Yes	Yes	Yes	5
Leenaars 2011[110]	Yes	Yes	Yes	Can't tell; detailed results of study selection not reported, no reasons for exclusions described.	No	No validity assessment.	No	No	Can't tell; data not reported for all studies.	2
Muralidharan 2009[111]	Yes	Yes	Yes	Yes	Yes	Yes	Yes	Yes	Yes	7
National Collaborating Centre for Mental Health 2005[100]	Yes	Yes	Yes	Yes	Yes	Yes	Yes	Yes	Yes	7
Newton 2010[112]	Yes	Yes	Yes	Yes	Yes	Yes	Yes	Yes	Yes	7
Pharaoh 2010[113]	Yes	Yes	Yes	Yes	Yes	Yes	Yes	Yes	Yes	7
Robinson 2011[93]	Yes	Yes	Yes	Can't tell; numbers of exclusions reported at each stage, but reasons not reported.	Yes	No; reported results of validity assessment in table and paragraph, but did not appear to account for variation in synthesis.	Yes	No; only 1 comparison with >1 study; and did not combine data and did not explain reasons for this.	Yes	4

Author Year of systematic review	Search methods reported	Comprehensive search	Inclusion criteria reported	Selection bias avoided	Validity criteria reported	Validity assessed appropriately	Methods used to combine studies reported	Findings combined appropriately	Conclusions supported by data	Overall scientific quality (higher score is better)
Sakinofsky 2007 (Parts 1 & 2) [94,95]	Partially; start date provided, but no end date.	Yes; several databases were used.	Can't tell; RCTs were the main focus but of necessity, it also considered other categories of investigations of the outcome of treatment.	No; no information related to number of articles found, included, and excluded.	No; did not describe criteria used to differentiate between good and deficiencies.	Yes; critical assessment of the quality of design, conduct and analysis of the studies was performed and reported according to authors' constructed schema of level of evidence.	Yes	Yes; report of findings follow simplified scheme of evidence constructed by authors.	Yes	4
Shek 2010 [114]	Yes	Yes; only searched one database, though this database combines multiple other databases.	Yes	Yes	Yes	Yes	Yes	Yes	Yes	7
Shekelle 2009 [14] & Bagley 2010 [103]	Yes	Yes	Yes	Yes	Yes	Yes	Yes	Yes	Yes	7
Soomro 2008 [96]	Yes	No; no hand-searching, reference list searching, or asking experts noted.	Yes	No	Yes	Yes	No	Yes	Yes	4
State of Victoria Department of Health 2010 [115]	Yes	No; no hand-searching, reference list searching, or asking experts noted.	Yes	Yes	Yes	Yes	Yes	Can't tell.	Yes	6
Takada 2010 [116]	Yes	No; no hand-searching, reference list searching, or asking experts noted.	Yes	Yes	Yes	Yes	No	No	No	3
Williams 2009 [98] & Williams 2009 [99]	Yes	Yes	Yes	Yes; study flow diagram in Pediatrics publication,[99] reasons for exclusion for individual trials provided in Evidence Report.[98]	Yes	Yes; excluded poor quality studies.	Yes	Yes; did not conduct meta-analyses due to heterogeneity	Yes	7

APPENDIX N. DATA ABSTRACTION OF PRIMARY STUDIES OBTAINED FROM GOOD QUALITY SYSTEMATIC REVIEWS RELATED TO PSYCHOTHERAPY

Author Year of systematic review	Time period and databases searched in systematic review	Eligibility criteria in systematic review	Study designs of eligible studies	Countries included in eligible studies	Sample size in eligible studies	Population in eligible studies	Interventions in eligible studies	Main results of eligible studies
Abbass 2009[102]	CCDANCTR-Studies, CCDANCTR-References; CENTRAL, MEDLINE, CIHAHL, EMBASE, PsycINFO, DARE, Biological Abstracts: database inception–April 2005	All RCTs in which short-term psychodynamic psychotherapies was compared with wait-list controls, minimal treatment controls which had been designated as psychological "placebo treatments," and treatments as usual; adult outpatients with common mental disorders (excluding psychotic disorders)	No eligible RCTs	No eligible RCTs	No eligible RCTs	No eligible RCTs	No eligible RCTs	No eligible RCTs
Binks 2011[104]	Medline: 1966–January 2003; PsycINFO: 1872–December 2002; CCRCT: to October 2002; EMBASE: 1980–January 2003; and 21 additional specialist databases	Clinical RCTs with or without blinding involving psychological treatments (behavioral, cognitive-behavioral, psychodynamic, and psychoanalytic) for adults with a diagnosis of borderline personality disorder	No eligible RCTs	No eligible RCTs	No eligible RCTs	No eligible RCTs	No eligible RCTs	No eligible RCTs
Dieterich 2010[106]	Cochrane Schizophrenia Group Trials Registry: database inception–February 2009	Randomized clinical trials focused on people with severe mental illness ages 18–65 years; community care setting; intensive case management (ICM) compared to non-ICM or standard care	No eligible RCTs	No eligible RCTs	No eligible RCTs	No eligible RCTs	No eligible RCTs	No eligible RCTs
Dubicka 2010[87]	PsycINFO, MEDLINE, Cochrane databases: January 1980–March 2009	RCTs predominantly including adolescents aged 11–18 years with a DSM-IV defined episode of depression where CBT was combined with a newer generation antidepressant and compared with antidepressant treatment without CBT	No eligible RCTs	No eligible RCTs	No eligible RCTs	No eligible RCTs	No eligible RCTs	No eligible RCTs
Irving 2010[107]	Cochrane Schizophrenia Group's Register of Trials: 1998–January 2006; additional searches in past versions of this review	RCTs and quasi-RCTs; patients with schizophrenia or other serious mental illness presenting to or referred to a social/psychiatric/ nursing service because they were experiencing a psychosocial crisis, however defined (excluded people in crisis with drug-induced psychosis or in a depressive crisis)	No eligible RCTs	No eligible RCTs	No eligible RCTs	No eligible RCTs	No eligible RCTs	No eligible RCTs
Kavanagh 2009[108]	MEDLINE, CINAHL, EMBASE, The Cochrane Library, PSYCINFO, ERIC, SOCIAL SCIENCE CITATION INDEX, ASSIA, Trials Register of Public Health Interventions (TROPHI), Database of Public Health Effectiveness Reviews (DOPHER), C2 SPECTR, PSITRI: Time period not reported	RCTs published from 1996 onwards in the English language that at least measured depression, anxiety, or suicidality following an intervention based on cognitive behavioral techniques delivered within secondary schools to young people aged 11–19	No eligible RCTs	No eligible RCTs	No eligible RCTs	No eligible RCTs	No eligible RCTs	No eligible RCTs
Muralidharan 2009[111]	CINAHL, CENTRAL, Schizophrenia Groups Register, EMBASE, MEDLINE, PsycINFO: database inception–January 2006	Relevant RCTs and quasi-RCTs; people with the diagnosis of serious mental illness (including "serious/chronic mental illness" or "psychotic illness"), however diagnosed	No eligible RCTs	No eligible RCTs	No eligible RCTs	No eligible RCTs	No eligible RCTs	No eligible RCTs

Suicide Prevention Interventions and Referral/Follow-up Services: A Systematic Review

Author Year of systematic review	Time period and databases searched in systematic review	Eligibility criteria in systematic review	Study designs of eligible studies	Countries included in eligible studies	Sample size in eligible studies	Population in eligible studies	Interventions in eligible studies	Main results of eligible studies
National Collaborating Centre for Mental Health 2005[100]	MEDLINE, EMBASE, PsycINFO, Cochrane Library: Inception to September 2004	RCTs of depressed participants aged 5-18 treated with CBT, CBT+separate parenting sessions, interpersonal psychotherapy, psychoanalytic/psychodynamic child psychotherapy, self-modeling, relaxation, social skills training, family therapy, guided self-help, or control enhancement training, and that reported remission, symptom levels, functional status or discontinuation from treatment for any reason outcomes.	No eligible RCTs	No eligible RCTs	No eligible RCTs	No eligible RCTs	No eligible RCTs	No eligible RCTs
Newton 2010[112]	MEDLINE, EMBASE, CCRCT, CDSR, Health Technology Assessment Database, DARE, Academic Search Elite, PsycINFO: 1985-October 2009; and 4 additional specialist databases	Experimental or quasi-experimental designs; mental health-based, suicide prevention-focused intervention initiated in the ED or immediately after ED discharge through direct referral/enrollment; children and adolescents (≤18 years), or their parents or ED personnel; ≥1 clinically relevant primary outcome	No eligible RCTs	No eligible RCTs	No eligible RCTs	No eligible RCTs	No eligible RCTs	No eligible RCTs
Pharaoh 2010[113]	Cochrane Schizophrenia Group Trials Register: to September 2008	Relevant RCTs or quasi-RCTs; studies where most (>75%) families included at least one member with a diagnosis of schizophrenia and/or schizoaffective disorder	No eligible RCTs	No eligible RCTs	No eligible RCTs	No eligible RCTs	No eligible RCTs	No eligible RCTs
Shek 2010[114]	Cochrane Schizophrenia Group Trials Register: to May 2009	Relevant RCTs; people aged 18-65 years and suffering from illness such as schizophrenia, schizophrenia-like disorders, and bipolar disorder (excluding acutely ill patients)	No eligible RCTs	No eligible RCTs	No eligible RCTs	No eligible RCTs	No eligible RCTs	No eligible RCTs
Shekelle 2009[14] & Bagley 2010[103]	MEDLINE, Cochrane Library, PsycINFO: June 2005-May 2008	English language; suicide or suicide attempt outcomes; no mental health interventions such as psychotherapy or pharmacotherapy unless they included Veterans	One RCT: Unutzer 2006	US	1,801	Non-Veteran/ military; no other data reported	Collaborative care model including case management in a primary care setting	No suicides in either treatment or control group
State of Victoria Department of Health 2010[115]	MEDLINE, EMBASE, AMED, PsycINFO: January 1997-February 2009	English language; human; suicide related outcome; sample size ≥6; no duplication; emergency department or other acute care setting	No eligible RCTs	No eligible RCTs	No eligible RCTs	No eligible RCTs	No eligible RCTs	No eligible RCTs
Williams 2009[98] & Williams 2009[99]	DARE, CDSR, MEDLINE, PsycINFO: 1998-May 2006	Patients aged 7-18 years with MDD or depression NOS; primary care setting, school-based clinics; English language only; excluded poor quality studies	No eligible RCTs	No eligible RCTs	No eligible RCTs	No eligible RCTs	No eligible RCTs	No eligible RCTs

APPENDIX O. SUMMARY OF SYSTEMATIC REVIEW RESULTS RELATED TO PSYCHOTHERAPY FROM GAYNES ET AL., MANN ET AL., AND NICE REVIEWS[9-11]

	Gaynes 2004[9]	Mann 2005[10]	NICE 2011[11]
Overall conclusions	The poor generalizability of the studies makes the overall strength of evidence fair, at best, while the results are mixed. Although some trends suggest incremental benefit from several interventions, no consistent statistically significant effects have emerged for interventions for which more than one study has been done.	Interventions need more evidence of efficacy.	Compared with usual care, there was insufficient evidence to determine clinical effects between interventions and routine care in the reduction of the proportion of patients who repeated self-harm. Thus, no conclusions could be made regarding psychosocial interventions on reduction of repetitions of self-harm. For the outcome of suicide, no conclusions could be drawn due to the small evidence base.
Scope			
Search dates	1966-October 2002	1966-June 2005	Up to January 2011
Populations included	Population of interest was primary care patients with previously unidentified suicide risk. Included RCTs were conducted in high-risk groups as identified by a deliberate self-harm episode, diagnosis of borderline personality disorder, or admission to a psychiatric unit.	Not specified	Adults, children, and young people with previous self-harm behavior
Interventions included	Pharmacotherapy, psychotherapy, referral/follow-up	Pharmacotherapy, psychotherapy, referral/follow-up	Pharmacotherapy, psychotherapy, referral/follow-up
Suicide-related outcomes included	Suicide completions, suicide attempts	Completed and attempted suicide	Primary outcome was repetition of self-harm; also included suicide outcomes.
Settings/countries included	Primary or specialty care settings; no exclusions based on country.	Included settings not specified; no exclusions based on country.	No exclusions by country
Other exclusion criteria	Clinical trials targeting patients with chronic psychotic illnesses; studies without adequate comparison groups.	No additional exclusion criteria specified.	
Main results: Psychotherapy			
Any psychological therapy (including problem-solving therapy, CBT, and psychodynamic therapy)			10 studies were combined, though study heterogeneity suggests that results should be interpreted with caution. Repetition of self-harm (up to 6 months, 2 studies): Less people from the treatment group had a repetition of self-harm compared with the TAU group; low quality. Repetition of self-harm (6 to 12 months, 5 studies): Less people from the treatment group had a repetition of self-harm compared with the TAU group; moderate quality. Repetition of self-harm (more than 12 months, 2 studies): Less people from the treatment group had a repetition of self-harm compared with the TAU group; low quality. Repetition of self-harm (at last follow-up, 9 studies): There was a statistically significant 24% reduction in chance of repetition in the treatment group compared with TAU; low quality.
Cognitive behavioral counseling/cognitive therapy	No significant difference in repeated suicidal behavior in one cohort study.	Cognitive therapy halved the reattempt rate in suicide attempters in one RCT.	Manual Assisted Cognitive Treatment: One study showed a non-significant reduction in self-harm, another showed a significant reduction. Results should be interpreted with caution due to study limitations.

	Gaynes 2004[9]	Mann 2005[10]	NICE 2011[11]
DBT	One RCT showed a reduction in repetition of deliberate self-harm in female veterans with borderline personality disorder.	Reduced suicidal behavior in people with borderline personality disorder.	DBT: The evidence showed some benefit in reducing rates of self-harm.
Intensive care plus outreach		Fewer suicide attempts.	
Interpersonal psychotherapy	Patients in therapy group were less likely to have a repeated episode of deliberate self-harm.	Fewer suicide attempts.	
Outpatient day hospitalization	No difference between groups.		
Problem-solving therapy	Meta-analysis of 5 studies showed a trend toward decreasing repetition of deliberate self-harm.	Fewer suicide attempts.	
Psychoanalytically oriented partial hospitalization	Fewer patients in the treatment group had attempted suicide at 36-month follow-up.	Reduced suicidal behavior in people with borderline personality disorder.	
Transference focused psychotherapy			Transference focused psychotherapy vs treatment by community psychotherapists: Significantly fewer attempted suicides in transference focused therapy group, but no difference in reduction of self-harm in either group. Results should be interpreted with caution due to study limitations.
Video education plus family therapy		No benefit in terms of re-attempt rate when compared to standard care.	
Main results: Comparative effectiveness of different types of therapy			
Home vs outpatient problem-solving therapy			No significant difference in repetition of self-harm in the year following treatment entry.
Inpatient behavior therapy vs inpatient insight-oriented therapy	No difference between groups.		Insufficient evidence to determine clinical differences between groups for repetition of self-harm.
Interpersonal problem-solving skills training vs brief problem-oriented therapy			Insufficient evidence to determine clinical differences between groups for repetition of self-harm. No suicides in either group.
Long-term therapy vs short-term therapy	No difference between groups.		Insufficient evidence to determine clinical differences between groups for repetition of self-harm.
Same therapist (continuity of care) vs different therapist (change of care)	No benefit for continuity of care.		Limited evidence suggesting that there was a clinically significant difference favoring different therapist over same therapist on reducing the likelihood of repetition of self-harm.

APPENDIX P. DESCRIPTION OF PRIMARY OUTCOMES AND INTENT TO TREAT SUICIDAL SELF-DIRECTED VIOLENCE FOR PSYCHOTHERAPY STUDIES

Study, Year	Designed to treat suicide? (yes/no/unclear)	N	Outcome definition	Results
Bateman 2008[17]	Yes; primary outcome was number of suicide attempts.	41	Suicidal behavior: 1) deliberate, 2) life-threatening, 3) resulted in medical intervention, and 4) medical assessment consistent with a suicide attempt. Self-harm: 1) deliberate, 2) resulted in visible tissue damage, and 3) nursing or medical intervention required.	Any suicide attempt: MBT=5/22 (23%) vs TAU=14/19 (74%); $\chi2$ (df=1)=8.7, P=0.003; effect size d=2.0 (95% CI, 1.4 to 4.9) Mean total number of suicide attempts (SD): MBT=0.05 (0.9) vs TAU=0.52 (0.48); U=73, z=3.9, P=0.00004; effect size d=1.4 (95% CI, 1.3 to 1.5)
Bateman 2009[37]	Yes; primary outcome declared prior to the study was the proportion of each group without severe parasuicidal behavior as indicated by: 1) suicide attempt, 2) life-threatening self-harm, or 3) hospital admission.	134	Suicidal behavior: 1) deliberate, 2) life-threatening, 3) resulted in medical intervention, and 4) medical assessment consistent with a suicide attempt. Self-harm: 1) deliberate, 2) resulted in visible tissue damage, and 3) nursing or medical intervention required. Outcomes assessed at 6, 12, and 18 months	Life-threatening suicide attempts: (A) Proportion with episode=N/%; (B) Average count=Mean(SD) After 6 months: MBT=(A) 37/52.1%, (B) 0.62 (0.74) vs SCM=(A) 33/52.4%, (B) 0.70 (0.81) After 12 months: MBT=(A) 23/32.4%, (B) 0.36 (0.57) vs SCM=(A) 30/47.6%, (B) 0.60 (0.77) After 18 months: MBT=(A) 2/2.8%, (B) 0.03 (0.17) vs SCM=(A) 16/25.4%, (B) 0.32 (0.62) Proportion with episode analysis: Wald $\chi2$ (df=3):76.21, P<0.001 Change over time=OR 0.41 (95% CI, 0.30 to 0.57); Group effect over time=OR 0.37 (95% CI, 0.21 to 0.62) At 12 months=RR 0.68 (95% CI, 0.44 to 1.04) In last 6 months=RR 0.11 (95% CI, 0.02 to 0.46) End of treatment difference= d=0.65 (95% CI, 0.58 to 0.73) Average count analysis: Wald $\chi2$ (df=3):212.56, P<0.001 Change over time=IRR 0.70 (95% CI, 0.62 to 0.80) Group effect over time=IRR 0.63 (95% CI, 0.53 to 0.75) Severe self-harm incidents: (A) Proportion with episode=N/%; (B) Average count=Mean (SD) After 6 months: MBT=(A) 53/74.6%, (B) 2.61 (3.08) vs SCM=(A) 37/58.7%, (B) 1.79 (2.62) After 12 months: MBT=(A) 26/36.6%, (B) 1.30 (2.47) vs SCM=(A) 37/58.7%, (B) 1.73 (2.27) After 18 months: MBT=(A) 17/23.9%, (B) 0.38 (0.83) vs SCM=(A) 27/42.9%, (B) 1.66 (2.86) Proportion with episode analysis: Wald $\chi2$ (df=3):62.77, P<0.001 Change over time=OR 0.49(95% CI, 0.35 to 0.69); Group effect over time=OR 0.39 (95% CI, 0.23 to 0.66) First 6 months: RR 1.27 (95% CI, 0.99 to 1.63) 6 to 18 months: RR NR, but "MBT showed steeper decline" In last 6 months=RR 0.55 (95% CI, 0.33 to 0.92) End of treatment difference= d=0.62 (95% CI, 0.28 to 0.97) Average count analysis: Wald $\chi2$ (df=3):224.11, P<0.001 Change over time=IRR 0.74 (95% CI, 0.65 to 0.85) Group effect over time=IRR 0.69 (95% CI, 0.59 to 0.82)

Study, Year	Designed to treat suicide? (yes/no/unclear)	N	Outcome definition	Results
Blum 2008[39]	Yes; secondary outcome measures included suicide attempts and self-harm acts.	165	Data on suicide attempts and self-harm acts were collected at 1, 3, 6, 9 and 12 months. Outcome criteria were not defined.	Not reported separately by treatment group: Suicide attempts: 24 (22.2%), median number of attempts was 1.75 per year, and the mean was 2.60 Self-harm acts: 56 (45.2%), the median number of acts was 9.8 per year, and the mean was 16.6 Cox proportional hazards analysis: treatment group was not associated with time to first suicide attempt ($\chi2<0.1$, df=1, p=0.994) or first self-harm act ($\chi2<0.1$, df=1, p=0.902)
Comtois 2011[47]	Yes; the Suicide Attempt and Self-Injury Count was an outcome measure.	32	Suicide attempts and self-inflicted injuries were categorized using the Suicide Attempt and Self-Injury Count SASI-C (Linehan 1996) at all follow-up assessments conducted at 2, 4, 6 and 12 months.	2 months: mean (SD) Suicide attempts/self-inflicted injuries: CAMS=N/A vs E-CAU=5.5 (7.8) ED admissions: CAMS=N/A vs E-CAU=0.5 (0.7) Behavioral health ED admissions only: CAMS=N/A vs E-CAU=1.1 (0.6) Number of inpatient days: CAMS=N/A vs E-CAU=4.0 (5.7) 4 months: mean (SD) Suicide attempts/self-inflicted injuries: CAMS=0.0 (0.0) vs E-CAU=0.8 (1.8) ED admissions: CAMS=0.4 (0.5) vs E-CAU=0.4 (0.7) Behavioral health ED admissions only: CAMS=0.1 (0.4) vs E-CAU=0.4 (0.7) Number of inpatient days: CAMS=1.4 (2.5) vs E-CAU=1.0 (2.3) 6 months: mean (SD) Suicide attempts/self-inflicted injuries: CAMS=0.2 (0.4) vs E-CAU=0.0 (0.0) ED admissions: CAMS=0.4 (0.5) vs E-CAU=0.2 (0.4) Behavioral health ED admissions only: CAMS=0.2 (0.4) vs E-CAU=0.2 (0.4) Number of inpatient days: CAMS=3.5 (7.0) vs E-CAU=1.3 (4.6) 12 months: mean (SD) Suicide attempts/self-inflicted injuries: CAMS=1.2 (3.9) vs E-CAU=3.3 (7.6) ED admissions: CAMS=0.4 (0.8) vs E-CAU=1.0 (2.4) Behavioral health ED admissions only: CAMS=0.2 (0.4) vs E-CAU=0.6 (1.6) Number of inpatient days: CAMS=1.4 (4.5) vs E-CAU=3.2 (8.0)
Davidson 2006[40]	Yes; occurrence of suicidal acts was a primary outcome.	106	Suicidal acts over 6 years, recorded using the Acts of Deliberate Self-Harm Inventory, which requires fulfillment of all 3 of the following criteria: 1) deliberate, 2) life threatening, and 3) the act resulted in medical intervention or intervention would have been warranted.	0-12 months (N=101) Subjects with suicidal acts: CBT= 18 (37%) vs TAU= 21 (46%). OR= 0.77 (95% CI ; 0.29 to 2.01) Mean episodes of suicidal acts (SD): CBT= 0.61 (0.95) vs TAU= 1.02 (2.14); adjusted Mean Difference (aMD)= −0.36 (95% CI, −0.83 to 0.13) 0-24 months (N=102) Subjects with suicidal acts: CBT= 23 (43%) vs TAU= 26 (54%). OR= 0.78 (95% CI ; 0.30 to 1.98) Mean episodes of suicidal acts (SD): CBT= 0.87 (1.47) vs TAU= 1.73 (3.11); aMD= −0.91 (95% CI, −1.67 to −0.15) 0-6 years (N=76) Subjects with suicidal acts: CBT= 56% (n = 24/43) vs TAU= 73% (n = 24/33); aOR = 0.37 (95% CI; 0.10 to 1.38) Mean episodes of suicidal acts (SD): CBT= 1.88 (3.19) vs TAU= 3.03 (4.16); aMD (TAU-CBT) = 1.26 (95% CI, -0.06 to 2.58)

Study, Year	Designed to treat suicide? (yes/no/unclear)	N	Outcome definition	Results
De Leo 2007[45]	No; outcomes were psychopathology, life functioning, suicidality (Scale for Suicidal Ideation), and satisfaction with services.	60 (22 completed 12 months of treatment)	Questions on functioning in life domains, health service use, and professional contacts determined in structured interviews with trained clinical psychologists, who performed the examinations (including self-report scales) at 6-monthly intervals; the first being immediately following discharge.	No suicides in the 12-month follow-up period. Self-harming behaviors (ICM vs TAU) 6 months: 3/14 (21.4%) vs 1/8 (12.4%) 12 months: 2/14 (14.3%) vs 2/8 (25.0%) P-values not reported
Diamond 2010[46]	No; suicidal ideation specified as an outcome, but not behaviors.	66	Clinical status monitored weekly using the SIQ-JR and BDI-II, administered either face-to-face (ABFT) or over the phone (EUC). Definition of "low lethality suicide attempts" not reported.	Low lethality suicide attempts: ABFT=11% (4/35); EUC=22% (7/31); p not reported
Donaldson 2005[48]	Yes; Structured adolescent and parent follow-up interviews assessed incidents of further suicidal behaviors.	39	Outcome measures were administered 3 months (end of active treatment) and 6 months (end of maintenance).	N=31 Reattempts at 6 months: SBT=26.7% (4/15) vs SRT=12.5% (2/16); χ^2=1.00 The difference in rates of suicide reattempts among those taking (n = 6/6) vs not taking (n = 0/25) medication was statistically significant: χ^2=7.95, P < .05
Green 2011[44]	No; primary outcome was frequency of episodes of self-harm; suicidal intent is not specified.	366	Primary outcome was the frequency of episodes of self-harm (includes non-suicidal self-harm).	3 episodes of self-harm resulting in severe physical injury (2 usual care, 1 group therapy). No suicides or other deaths.

Study, Year	Designed to treat suicide? (yes/no/unclear)	N	Outcome definition	Results
Hatcher 2011[36]	Yes; the primary outcome was presentation to hospital with self-harm in the year after the index attempt.	1094	Obtained from the New Zealand Health Information Service details of hospital contacts throughout New Zealand in the year after the index attempt. Data obtained from the National Minimum Dataset kept by the New Zealand Health Information Service, which contains routinely collected information on all public and private hospital discharges in New Zealand.	Consenting Patients Participants re-presenting to hospital for self-harm; PST+TAU vs TAU: All index episodes (N=253 vs 299): 14.2% vs 17.1%; RR=0.17 (95% CI -0.24 to 0.44); P=0.43 Index episode is first self-harm episode (N=137 vs 169): 13.9% vs 8.9%; RR=-0.56 (95% CI -1.96 to 0.18); P=0.23 Index episode is repeat episode (N=116 vs 130): 14.7% vs 27.7%; RR=0.47 (95% CI 0.11 to 0.69); P=0.02; NNT=8 Participants with self-reported self-harm; PST+TAU vs TAU: All index episodes (N=186 vs 226): 27.4% vs 32.7%; RR=0.16 (95% CI -0.13 to 0.38); P=0.29 Index episode is first self-harm episode (N=98 vs 122): 25.5% vs 20.5%; RR= -0.25 (95% CI -1.03 to 0.24); P=0.47 Index episode is repeat episode (N=88 vs 104): 29.5% vs 47.1%; RR=0.37 (95% CI 0.08 to 0.57); P=0.02; NNT=6 Time to re-presentation to hospital, days : median; PST+TAU vs TAU: All index episodes: 56 vs 83; HR=0.81 (95% CI 0.53 to 1.25); P=0.92 Index episode is first self-harm episode: 62 vs 75; HR=1.62 (95% CI 0.82 to 3.18); P=0.16 Index episode is repeat episode: 45 vs 104; HR=0.47 (95% CI 0.26 to 0.85); P=0.01 All Patients Participants re-presenting to hospital for self-harm; PST+TAU vs TAU: All index episodes (N=522 vs 572): 13.4% vs 14.1%; RR=0.05 (95% CI -0.28 to 0.30); P=0.79 Index episode is first self-harm episode (N=314 vs 360): 13.4% vs 9.4%; RR=-0.42 (95% CI -1.17 to 0.08); P=0.37 Index episode is repeat episode (N=208 vs 212): 13.5% vs 22.1%; RR=0.39 (95% CI 0.07 to 0.60); P=0.03; NNT=12 Time to re-presentation to hospital, days : median; PST+TAU vs TAU: All index episodes: 74 vs 75; HR=0.98 (95% CI 0.71 to 1.36); P=0.92 Index episode is first self-harm episode: 74 vs 61; HR=1.55 (95% CI 0.98 to 2.48); P=0.06 Index episode is repeat episode: 80 vs 114; HR=0.58 (95% CI 0.36 to 0.94); P=0.03
Hazell 2009[49]	Yes, the primary outcome measure was repetition of self-harm.	72	Defined as any intentional self-inflicted injury (including poisoning) irrespective of the apparent purpose of the behavior, based on an interview-based assessment of suicide behavior (Kerfoot 1992, Linehan 1999).	Repetition of Deliberate Self-harm by 6 months: GT = 88% (30/34); RC = 68% (23/34); p = 0.04 Repetition of Deliberate Self-harm in interval of 6 to 12 months: GT = 88% (30/34); RC = 71% (24/34); p = 0.07
Linehan 2006[38]	Yes; main outcome was suicidal behavior.	111	The Suicide Attempt Self-Injury Interview (Seligman 2006) measured the topography, suicide intent, and medical severity of each suicide attempt and nonsuicidal self-injury. Assessments completed at 4-month intervals during the 12-month treatment and 12 months of post-treatment follow-up periods by blinded, independent clinical assessors with master's or doctoral degrees.	Median suicides (interquartile range): DBT=0 (0 to 0) vs CTBE=0 (0 to 1) Suicide attempts: DBT=23.1% vs CTBE=46%, P=0.01, HR=2.66 (95% CI not reported); P=0.005), NNT=4.24 (95% CI, 2.40 to 18.07) Nonambivalent suicide attempts: DBT=5.8% vs CTBE=13.3%, P=0.18, NNT=13.3 (95% CI, 5.28 to 25.41) Suicide attempts per period: Significantly fewer in the DBT group across the 2 years when controlling for number of suicide attempts during the pretreatment year (F1,94=3.20, P=.04, MMANOVA) Mean proportions of suicide attempters per period: DBT=6.2% (95% CI, 3.1% to 11.7%) vs CTBE=12.2% (95% CI, 7.1% to 20.3%)

Study, Year	Designed to treat suicide? (yes/no/unclear)	N	Outcome definition	Results
McMain 2009[42]	Yes; the primary outcome measures were frequency and severity of suicidal and nonsuicidal self-injurious behavior episodes.	180	Assessed every 4 months by the Suicide Attempt Self-Injury Interview (M.M. Linehan et al., unpublished 1983 manuscript).	Deaths by suicide: None Mean number of suicidal and self-injurious episodes (SD): OR 0.92 (P=0.76) 4 months: DBT=10.60 (20.96) vs GPM=14.02 (43.87) 8 months: DBT=8.94 (19.07) vs GPM=11.44 (37.59) 12 months: DBT=4.29 (9.32) vs GPM=12.87 (51.45)
Stewart 2009[50]	Yes; one of the outcomes was re-presentation to the hospital for a suicide attempt.	32 (sample size is unclear)	Hospital chart audits recorded re-presentation to the hospital for suicide attempts.	Average number of suicide attempts: CBT: 0.22 (SD=0.64) PST: 0.33 (SD=0.63) TAU: 0.22 (SD=0.50) No significant differences found for repetition of suicide attempts when PST group was compared to TAU (U=35, ns, r=0.13) and when CBT was compared to TAU (U=25, ns, r=0.32)
Tarrier 2006[51]	No; objective of the article is to report suicidal behavior outcomes, but suicide was not a primary outcome of the SoCRATES Trial.	278	Deaths for any reason identified from hospital and psychiatric notes. Suicides and possible suicides (where the death might have been intentional or accidental and the coroner ruled the death was accidental) were identified. Suicide ideation and behavior (combined) assessed by the non-accidental self-injury scale of the HoNOS (Health of the Nation Outcome Scales). Serious risk (score of 4) indicates suicidal attempts or deliberate self-harm. Assessed at 6 weeks, 3 months, and 18 months.	Over 18 months, there were 3 definite suicides (1.2%), 2 in the supportive counseling group and 1 in CBT group. 4 further deaths classified as accidental by the coroner (1 traffic accident, 1 fall from window, 1 in supportive counseling group, 1 in CBT group). 2 deaths by natural causes. Numbers too small for meaningful statistical analysis. On the HoNOS, there were no significant differences between the 3 treatment groups at any time point. Psychological treatment did not significantly reduce or worsen suicidal behavior compared to treatment as usual. There was a marked reduction in suicidal behavior after admission that would mask any potential treatment effect.
Unutzer 2006[52]	No; suicidal ideation specified as an outcome, but not behaviors.	1801	Primary outcome was suicidal ideation. No information on how deaths were ascertained.	117 participants died before the 24-month follow-up; 61 of them (52%) were in the intervention group. To the authors' knowledge, there were no suicides in either group during the 2-year study period.
Winter 2007[43]	Yes; primary outcome was suicidal ideation, but records from the Accident and Emergency departments involved in the study were also monitored for repeat episodes of self-harm in participants in the 3 years following their initial presentation.	40	Primary outcomes were measure of suicidal ideation and depression. For assessment of self-harm, records from the Accident and Emergency departments involved in the study were monitored for repeat episodes of self-harm in the 3 years following their initial presentation.	Repetition of deliberate self-harm, intervention vs control: At 1 year: 17% vs 36% (P=0.12) At 3 years: 35% vs 53% (P=0.18) At 5 years: 39% vs 58% (P=0.15) No repetition within 5 years: 61% vs 42% (P not reported) 3 of the episodes eventuated in suicide death (1 intervention, 2 control)

APPENDIX Q. DATA ABSTRACTION FOR PRIMARY STUDIES RELATED TO PSYCHOTHERAPY

Author, Year (Country):	Bateman 2008[117] (UK)
Population:	Adults with borderline personality disorder
Therapy 1:	MBT by partial hospitalization consists of 18-month individual and group psychotherapy in a partial hospital setting offered within a structured and integrated program provided by a supervised team. Expressive therapy using art and writing groups is included. Crises are managed within the team; medication is prescribed according to protocol by a psychiatrist working in the therapy program. The understanding of behavior in terms of underlying mental states forms a common thread running across all aspects of treatment. The focus of therapy is on the patient's moment-to-moment state of mind. The patient and therapist collaboratively try to generate alternative perspectives to the patient's subjective experience of himself or herself and others by moving from validating and supportive interventions to exploring the therapy relationship itself as it suggests alternative understanding. This psychodynamic therapy is manualized (17) and in many respects overlaps with transference-focused psychotherapy. At the end of 18 months, the MBT by partial hospitalization patients were offered twice-weekly outpatient mentalizing group psychotherapy for a further 18 months,
Therapy 2:	Treatment as usual (TAU) consists of general psychiatric outpatient care with medication prescribed by the consultant psychiatrist, community support from mental health nurses, and periods of partial hospital and inpatient treatment as necessary but no specialist psychotherapy. After 18 months, the TAU group continued with general psychiatric care with psychotherapy but not MBT if recommended by the consultant psychiatrist.
Medication regimen:	Not specified
Setting:	Partial hospital program
Therapist characteristics:	Generic mental health professionals
Treatment duration:	36 months
N:	41: MBT=22, TAU=19
Mean age, % female, race (variance):	Age (SD): MBT=30.3 years (5.86), TAU=33.3 years (6.60) % Female: MBT=68%, TAU=47% Race NR
Other clinical characteristics:	Not reported
Concomitant medications:	Medication years (SD) Antidepressants: MBT=1.1 (1.8) vs TAU=3.3 (2.3) F (df=1, 35)=11.6, $P= 0.002$; effect size 1.10 (95% CI, 0.45 to 1.70) Antipsychotics: MBT= 0.16 (0.28) vs TAU= 3.1 (2.1); U=9.0, z=5.4, P=0.0000000005; effect size= 2.04 (95% CI, 1.60 to 2.50) Mood stabilizers: MBT=0.11 (0.26) vs TAU=1.8(2.1); U=105.0, z=3.2, P=0.001; effect size=1.17 (95% CI, 0.73 to 1.60) Three or more drugs (including hypnotics): MBT=0.02 (0.11) vs TAU=1.9 (1.9); U=58.5, z=4.6, P=0.0000009; effect size=1.45 (95% CI, 1.10 to 1.80).
Outcome assessment:	Number of suicide attempts over the whole of the 5-year postdischarge follow-up period. Suicidal behavior: 1) deliberate, 2) life-threatening, 3) resulted in medical intervention, and 4) medical assessment consistent with a suicide attempt. Self-harm: 1) deliberate, 2) resulted in visible tissue damage, and 3) nursing or medical intervention required.
Results:	Any suicide attempt: MBT=5/22 (23%) vs TAU=14/19 (74%); χ^2 (df=1)=8.7, P=0.003; effect size d=2.0 (95% CI, 1.4 to 4.9) Mean total number of suicide attempts (SD): MBT=0.05 (0.9) vs TAU=0.52 (0.48); U=73, z=3.9, P=0.00004; effect size d=1.4 (95% CI, 1.3 to 1.5)

Author, Year (Country):	Bateman 2009[37] (UK)
Population:	Adults with borderline personality disorder
Therapy 1:	MBT: Focused on helping patients reinstate mentalizing during a crisis via telephone contact and included: 1) once-weekly individual psychoanalytic psychotherapy; 2) thrice weekly group analytic psychotherapy (1 hour each); 3) once-a-week expressive therapy oriented toward psychodrama techniques (1 hour); and 4) a weekly community meeting (1 hour), all spread over 5 days. In addition, on a once-per-month basis, subjects had: 5) a meeting with the case administrator (1 hour); and 6) medication review by the resident psychiatrist.
Therapy 2:	SCM: Focused on support and problem solving, and included weekly combined individual and group psychotherapy and psychiatric review every 3 months. Therapy was based on a counseling model closest to a supportive approach with case management, advocacy support, and problem-oriented psychotherapeutic interventions.
Medication regimen:	The initial types and doses of medication were the same for both groups, and consisted of antidepressant and antipsychotic drugs prescribed as appropriate; polypharmacy was discouraged.
Setting:	Outpatient context in publicly-funded specialist personality disorder treatment center

Therapist characteristics:	Nonspecialist mental health practitioners
Treatment duration:	18 months
N:	134; MBT=71, SCM=63
Mean age, % female, race (variance):	Age, years: MBT=31.3 (SD=7.6); SCM=30.9 (SD=7.9) % female: MBT=80.3%, SCM=79.4% White British/European: MBT=76.1%, SCM=68.3% Black African/Afro-Caribbean: MBT=15.5%, SCM=20.6% Other Chinese/Turkish/Pakistani: MBT=8.5%, SCM=11.1%
Other clinical characteristics:	Rape: MBT=33.8% vs SCM=17.5% Drug use (> 4 times/week): MBT=40.8% vs 41.3% Suicide attempt past 6 months: MBT=74.6% vs 66.7% Current Axis I disorders: Major depressive disorder: MBT=57.7% vs SCM=54.0%; Depressive disorders include dysthymia: MBT=78.9% vs SCM=74.6%; Posttraumatic stress disorder: MBT=12.7% vs SCM=15.9%; any anxiety disorder: MBT=59.2% vs SCM=63.5%; Any substance use disorder: MBT=54.9% vs SCM=52.4%; Any eating disorder: MBT=28.2% vs SCM=27.0%; Somatoform disorder: MBT=11.3% vs SCM=14.3%
Concomitant medications:	Not reported
Outcome assessment:	Suicidal behavior: 1) deliberate, 2) life-threatening, 3) resulted in medical intervention, and 4) medical assessment consistent with a suicide attempt. Self-harm: 1) deliberate, 2) resulted in visible tissue damage, and 3) nursing or medical intervention required. Outcomes assessed at 6, 12, and 18 months.
Results:	Life-threatening suicide attempts: (A) Proportion with episode=N/%: (B) Average count=Mean(SD) After 6 months: MBT=(A) 37/52.1%, (B) 0.62 (0.74) vs SCM=(A) 33/52.4%, (B) 0.70 (0.81) After 12 months: MBT=(A) 23/32.4%, (B) 0.36 (0.57) vs SCM=(A) 30/47.6%, (B) 0.60 (0.77) After 18 months: MBT=(A) 2/2.8%, (B) 0.03 (0.17) vs SCM=(A) 16/25.4%, (B) 0.32 (0.62) Proportion with episode analysis: Wald χ^2 (df=3):76.21, P<0.001 Change over time=CR 0.41 (95% CI, 0.30 to 0.57); Group effect over time=OR 0.37 (95% CI, 0.21 to 0.62) At 12 months=RR 0.68 (95% CI, 0.44 to 1.04) In last 6 months=RR 0.11 (95% CI, 0.02 to 0.46) End of treatment difference=d=0.65 (95% CI, 0.58 to 0.73) Average count analysis: Wald χ^2 (df=3):212.56, P<0.001 Change over time=IRR 0.70 (95% CI, 0.62 to 0.80) Group effect over time=IRR 0.63 (95% CI, 0.53 to 0.75) Severe self-harm incidents: (A) Proportion with episode=N/%: (B) Average count=Mean(SD) After 6 months: MBT=(A) 53/74.6%, (B) 2.61(3.08) vs SCM=(A) 37/58.7%, (B) 1.79 (2.62) After 12 months: MBT=(A) 26/36.6%, (B) 1.30 (2.47) vs SCM=(A) 37/58.7%, (B) 1.73 (2.27) After 18 months: MBT=(A) 17/23.9%, (B) 0.38 (0.83) vs SCM=(A) 27/42.9%, (B) 1.66 (2.86) Proportion with episode analysis: Wald χ^2 (df=3):62.77, P<0.001 Change over time=OR 0.49(95% CI, 0.35 to 0.69); Group effect over time=OR 0.39 (95% CI, 0.23 to 0.66) First 6 months: RR 1.27 (95% CI, 0.99 to 1.63) 6 to 18 months: RR NR, but "MBT showed steeper decline" In last 6 months=RR 0.55 (95% CI, 0.33 to 0.92) End of treatment difference=d=0.62 (95% CI, 0.28 to 0.97) Average count analysis: Wald χ^2 (df=3):224.11, P<0.001 Change over time=IRR 0.74 (95% CI, 0.65 to 0.85) Group effect over time=IRR 0.69 (95% CI, 0.59 to 0.82)

Author, Year (Country):	Blum 2008[39] (US)
Population:	Adults with borderline personality disorder

Therapy 1:	Treatment as usual (TAU): Continuation of usual care, including individual psychotherapy, medication, and case management. Subjects received no instructions or advice about other pharmacologic or psychotherapeutic treatments.
Therapy 2	Systems Training for Emotional Predictability and Problem Solving (STEPPS) plus TAU: STEPPS is a manual-based group treatment program that combines cognitive behavioral elements with skills training and has the following three main components: 1) psychoeducation, 2) emotion management skills training, and 3) behavior management skills training. The program involves 20 2-hour weekly sessions with 2 co-facilitators who follow a detailed lesson plan that includes homework assignments. STEPPS is systems-based in that family members, significant others, and health care professionals are educated about borderline personality disorder and instructed how best to interact with their relative or friend with the disorder.
Medication regimen:	Not specified
Setting:	Outpatient, group sessions with the look and feel of a seminar. Exact setting not specified.
Therapist characteristics:	Administered by 2 of the authors of the study (Ms. Blum and Mr. St. John)
Treatment duration:	20 weeks
N:	165: STEPPS=93 vs TAU=72
Mean age, % female, race (variance):	Mean age, years (SD): 31.5 (9.5) 83% female 94% Caucasian 2% African American 3% Other
Other clinical characteristics:	73% past suicide attempts 73% current major depressive disorder 1.8% DSM-IV personality disorders
Concomitant medications:	2.3% psychotropic medication use
Outcome assessment:	Data on suicide attempts and self-harm acts were collected at 1, 3, 6, 9 and 12 months. Outcome criteria were not defined.
Results:	Not reported separately by treatment group: Suicide attempts: 24 (22.2%), median number of attempts was 1.75 per year, and the mean was 2.60 Self-harm acts: 56 (45.2%), the median number of acts was 9.8 per year, and the mean was 16.6 Cox proportional hazards analysis: treatment group was not associated with time to first suicide attempt (χ^2<0.1, df=1, p=0.994) or first self-harm act (χ^2<0.1, df=1, p=0.902)

Author, Year (Country):	BOSCOT Trial (Borderline Personality Disorder Study of Cognitive Therapy) (UK) Davidson 2006[40] – 1-year outcomes Davidson 2010[41] – 6-year outcomes
Population:	Aged between 18 and 65 years, met criteria for at least 5 items of the borderline personality disorder using the Structured Clinical Interview for DSM-IV Axis II Personality Disorders, and had received either in-patient psychiatric services or an assessment at accident and emergency services or an episode of deliberate self-harm (either suicidal act or self-mutilation) in the previous 12 months
Therapy 1:	Treatment as usual (TAU): Included a wide variety of resources such as inpatient and outpatient hospital services, including A&E services, community based services such as drop in centers, and primary and community care services (GP, practice nurse, Community Psychiatric Nurse, etc.).
Therapy 2:	CBT specific to Cluster B personality disorder was delivered in up to 30 sessions of CBT over 1 year, each session lasting an hour, plus TAU.
Medication regimen:	Not reported
Setting:	Within the National Health Service in the U.K
Therapist characteristics:	5 therapists provided CBT in the trial. 4 were registered mental nurses and one, an occupational therapist. 3 of the therapists had completed a 10-month CBT training course and had a certificate in cognitive therapy, and 1 therapist had received CBT training in psychosis. Only 1 therapist had no previous training in CBT but had experience of managing individuals with personality disorder.
Treatment duration:	1 year
N:	106: CBT=54 vs TAU=52

Mean age, % female, race (variance):	Mean age (SD, range): 31.9 (9.1; 18-57) 84% female 100% White
Other clinical characteristics:	Beck Depression Inventory II Total Score, mean (SD): 42.5 (11.2) Average number of years since first act of deliberate self-harm (SD): 14.8 (10.0)
Concomitant medications:	Not reported
Outcome assessment:	Suicidal acts over 6 years, recorded using the Acts of Deliberate Self-Harm Inventory, which requires fulfillment of all 3 of the following criteria: 1) deliberate, 2) life threatening, and 3) the act resulted in medical intervention or intervention would have been warranted.
Results:	0-12 months (N=101): Subjects with suicidal acts: CBT= 18 (37%) vs TAU= 21 (46%). OR= 0.77 (95% CI ; 0.29 to 2.01) Mean episodes of suicidal acts (SD): CBT= 0.61 (0.95) vs TAU= 1.02 (2.14); adjusted Mean Difference (aMD)= −0.36 (95% CI, −0.83 to 0.13) 0-24 months (N=102): Subjects with suicidal acts: CBT= 23 (43%) vs TAU= 26 (54%). OR= 0.78 (95% CI ; 0.30 to 1.98) Mean episodes of suicidal acts (SD): CBT= 0.87 (1.47) vs TAU= 1.73 (3.11); aMD= −0.91 (95% CI, −1.67 to −0.15) 0-6 years (N=76): Subjects with suicidal acts: CBT= 56% (n = 24/43) vs TAU= 73% (n = 24/33); aOR = 0.37 (95% CI, 0.10 to 1.38) Mean episodes of suicidal acts (SD): CBT= 1.88 (3.19) vs TAU= 3.03 (4.16); aMD (TAU-CBT) = 1.26 (95% CI, −0.06 to 2.58)

Author, Year (Country):	Comtois 2011[47] (US)
Population:	Adults with a recent suicide attempt or imminent risk who (a) did not have appropriate outpatient mental health treatment available for an appointment in the next 2 weeks; (b) a NDA and weekly outpatient follow-up was an appropriate disposition plan, and (c) the patient was sufficiently stable to be discharged home for a minimum of 24 hours prior to NDA appointment.
Therapy 1:	CAMS: Intervention developed by the second author that modifies how clinicians engage, assess, and treat suicidality. CAMS involves the use of a Suicide Status Form (SSF) to guide assessment, treatment planning, on-going tracking of risk, and outcome/disposition of care. The SSF involves quantitative and qualitative assessments and consideration of empirically-based risk factors. CAMS sessions are provided weekly, generally for 50-60 minutes. CAMS generally lasts from a minimum of 4 sessions up to approximately 12 sessions.
Therapy 2:	E-CAU: Intake with the psychiatrist or psychiatric nurse practitioner followed by 1–11 visits with a case manager and as needed medication management. Treatment ends in 1–3 months when the "crisis is resolved" with referral for primary care follow-up or, when there is an appropriate diagnosis and funding is available, additional mental health or substance abuse treatment. Care in the study was enhanced by funding equivalent clinician time in both conditions and clinicians in both conditions were asked to schedule a minimum of 4 sessions (i.e., the minimum number of sessions in CAMS).
Medication regimen:	Not reported
Setting:	Outpatient crisis intervention setting attached to Harborview Medical Center, a county-owned, safety net hospital focused on underserved and unfunded populations. Study treatment conditions were provided in the Crisis Intervention Service to which all Harborview next-day appointments are referred.
Therapist characteristics:	CAMS: 4 clinicians (1 case manager, 2 psychologists, and 1 psychiatry resident) provided treatment after participating in a 1-day didactic training by Dr. Jobes, the CAMS developer and reaching acceptable levels of adherence. E-CAU: Provided by case managers with average years since degree=27.5, SD53.5
Treatment duration:	Variable, minimum of 4 sessions
N:	32: CAMS=16 vs E-CAU-16
Mean age, % female, race (variance)	Mean age (SD, range)=36.8 years (10.1, 19-62) 62% women 66% Caucasian
Other clinical characteristics:	0 months: mean (SD) Suicide attempts/self-inflicted injuries: CAMS=3.0 (9.3) vs E-CAU=7.7 (24.5) ED admissions: CAMS=1.5 (1.2) vs E-CAU=1.6 (0.8) Behavioral health ED admissions only: CAMS=1.3 (1.1) vs E-CAU=1.1 (0.6) Number of inpatient days: CAMS=5.5 (5.4) vs E-CAU=7.0 (7.0)
Concomitant medications:	Not reported

Outcome assessment:	Suicide attempts and self-inflicted injuries were categorized using the Suicide Attempt and Self-Injury Count SASI-C (Linehan 1996) at all follow-up assessments conducted at 2, 4, 6 and 12 months.
Results:	2 months: mean (SD) Suicide attempts/self-inflicted injuries: CAMS=N/A vs E-CAU=5.5 (7.8) ED admissions: CAMS=N/A vs E-CAU=0.5 (0.7) Behavioral health ED admissions only: CAMS=N/A vs E-CAU=1.1 (0.6) Number of inpatient days: CAMS=N/A vs E-CAU=4.0 (5.7) 4 months: mean (SD) Suicide attempts/self-inflicted injuries: CAMS=0.0 (0.0) vs E-CAU=0.8 (1.8) ED admissions: CAMS=0.4 (0.5) vs E-CAU=0.4 (0.7) Behavioral health ED admissions only: CAMS=0.1 (0.4) vs E-CAU=0.4 (0.7) Number of inpatient days: CAMS=1.4 (2.5) vs E-CAU=1.0 (2.3) 6 months: mean (SD) Suicide attempts/self-inflicted injuries: CAMS=0.2 (0.4) vs E-CAU=0.0 (0.0) ED admissions: CAMS=0.4 (0.5) vs E-CAU=0.2 (0.4) Behavioral health ED admissions only: CAMS=0.2 (0.4) vs E-CAU=0.2 (0.4) Number of inpatient days: CAMS=3.5 (7.0) vs E-CAU=1.3 (4.6) 12 months: mean (SD) Suicide attempts/self-inflicted injuries: CAMS=1.2 (3.9) vs E-CAU=3.3 (7.6) ED admissions: CAMS=0.4 (0.8) vs E-CAU=1.0 (2.4) Behavioral health ED admissions only: CAMS=0.2 (0.4) vs E-CAU=0.6 (1.6) Number of inpatient days: CAMS=1.4 (4.5) vs E-CAU=3.2 (8.0)

Author, Year (Country):	De Leo 2007[45] (Australia)
Population:	Men ages 18 years and older with a current admission at the local psychiatric ward due to severe suicidal ideation and/or attempt as the main motive for hospitalization.
Therapy 1:	Intensive case management (ICM): Case managers from a community mental health service had weekly face-to-face sessions with participants; intervention based on the rehabilitation model described by Rapp and Kisthardt. Outreach provided in a variety of settings including home visits; frequent contact, with a minimum of one contact per week for 12 months; staff available outside appointment times but within regular work hours; client-focused approach tailored to each individual; emphasis on skills-building and problem solving, encourages client empowerment and independence; linkage to services; advocacy services; provision of individual and group psychotherapy and counseling services; 2 telephone calls a week from counselors collaborating with case managers.
Therapy 2:	Treatment as usual: Individual Program Plans, pharmacotherapy, referrals to general practitioners, psychologists, psychiatrists, rehabilitation services, and/or the routine level of case management but not telephone calls from counselors.
Medication regimen:	None.
Setting:	Community mental health service.
Therapist characteristics:	Qualified mental health professionals with specialist training in mental psychotherapeutic techniques (e.g., psychologist, psychiatric nurse).
Treatment duration:	Mean 49.75 weeks.
N:	60 (22 completed 12-month treatment: 14 ICM, 8 TAU)
Mean age, % female, race (variance):	ICM vs TAU: Median age 34 years (range 24-59) vs 37 years (range 19-62) 100% male Race not reported
Other clinical characteristics:	80% unipolar depression; 17% bipolar depression; 10% psychotic disorder; 8% substance abuse disorder; 2% other diagnosis; 44% comorbid diagnoses.
Concomitant medications:	Not reported
Outcome assessment:	Questions on functioning in life domains, health service use, and professional contacts determined in structured interviews with trained clinical psychologists, who performed the examinations (including self-report scales) at 6-monthly intervals; the first being immediately following discharge.

Results:	No suicides in the 12-month follow-up period. Self-harming behaviors (ICM vs TAU) 6 months: 3/14 (21.4%) vs 1/8 (12.4%) 12 months: 2/14 (14.3%) vs 2/8 (25.0%) P-values not reported

Author, Year (Country):	Diamond 2010[46] (US)
Population:	Suicidal adolescents (Suicidal Ideation Questionnaire (SIQJR) score > 31; Beck Depression Inventory (BDI-II) > 20) between the ages of 12 and 17, identified in primary care and emergency departments
Therapy 1:	Attention-Based Family Therapy (ABFT): Focuses on strengthening parent-adolescent attachment bonds using a process-oriented, emotion-focused semistructured treatment protocol conceptualized as 5 specific tasks: 1) Relational Reframe Task to strengthen relationships; 2) Adolescent Alliance Task to prepare adolescent to discuss core family conflicts with parents; 3) Parent Alliance Task to teach emotionally focused parenting skills; 4) Reattachment Task for families to practice new skills; and 5) Competency Task to promote adolescent autonomy.
Therapy 2:	Enhanced Usual Care (EUC): A facilitated referral process with ongoing clinical monitoring.
Medication regimen:	Antidepressant medication allowed if started ≥12 weeks before randomization.
Setting:	Department of Psychiatry at the Children's Hospital of Philadelphia (CHOP).
Therapist characteristics:	Seven Ph.D.- or M.S.N.-level therapists provided ABFT under supervision of Guy and Gary Diamond
Treatment duration:	24 weeks
N:	66
Mean age, % female, race (variance):	Mean age, years (SD): ABFT=15.11 (1.41) vs EUC=15.29 (1.83) % Female: ABFT=91.4% vs EUC=74.2% African American: ABFT=71.4% vs EUC= 77.4%
Other clinical characteristics:	Current psychiatric diagnoses, % patients Major depressive episode: ABFT=37.1% vs EUC=41.9% Dysthymia: ABFT=8.3% vs EUC=6.52% Any anxiety: ABFT=60.0% vs EUC=74.2% Externalizing disorder (ADHD, ODD, CD): ABFT=65% vs EUC=48% Clinical History, % patients Adolescent attempted suicide in the past: ABFT=61.3% vs EUC=62.9% Multiple attempts: ABFT=81.8% vs EUC=63.2% Past psychiatric hospitalization: ABFT=20.0% vs EUC=24.1% Taking antidepressant medicine: ABFT=8.6% vs EUC=10.3% Family history of suicide attempt: ABFT=30.3% vs EUC=34.3%
Concomitant medications:	Taking antidepressant medicine: ABFT 8.6% vs EUC=10.3%
Outcome assessment:	Clinical status monitored weekly using the SIQ-JR and BDI-II, administered either face-to-face (ABFT) or over the phone (EUC). Definition of "low lethality suicide attempts" not reported.
Results:	Low lethality suicide attempts: ABFT=11% (4/35); EUC=22% (7/31); p not reported

Author, Year (Country):	Donaldson 2005[48] (US)
Population:	Adolescents (12–17 years old) who presented to a general pediatric emergency department or inpatient unit of an affiliated child psychiatric hospital in the Northeast after a suicide attempt. Any intentional, nonfatal self-injury, regardless of medical lethality, was considered a suicide attempt if intent to die was indicated
Therapy 1:	Skills-Based Treatment (SBT): Focused on problem solving and affect management skills. Each session included an assessment of suicidality, skill education, and skill practice (both in-session and homework assignments). Participants were taught steps of effective problem solving and cognitive and behavioral strategies for affect management (e.g., cognitive restructuring, relaxation) and given homework assignments to assist in skill acquisition and generalization. The SBT included active and maintenance treatment phases. The active phase included 6 individual sessions and 1 adjunct family session administered during the first 3 months of treatment. The maintenance phase included 3 monthly sessions. At the therapist's discretion, 2 additional family sessions and 2 crisis sessions were available.

Therapy 2:	Supportive Relationship Treatment (SRT): Was adapted from the Supportive Relationship Treatment Manual of Brent and Kolko (1991). This treatment was supportive in nature and focused the adolescent's mood and behavior as well as factors that contribute to adolescent suicidal behavior. Sessions were unstructured and addressed reported symptoms and problems. Techniques included exploratory questioning, encouraging affect, connecting affect to events, and providing feedback about changes obtained in treatment. In contrast to SBT, specific skills were not taught and homework assignments were not given during any of the SRT sessions. The session protocol for SRT was identify to that of SBT (described above).
Medication regimen:	Not reported
Setting:	Not reported
Therapist characteristics:	7 therapists provided both treatments. 5 of the therapists held a doctorate in clinical psychology, 1 a master's degree in psychology, and 1 a master's degree in social work. Therapists received training in both approaches to allow for a crossed design
Treatment duration:	6 months
N:	39: SBT=21 vs SRT=18
Mean age, % female, race (variance):	Mean age (SD)=15.0 (1.7) 82% female 85% White 10% Hispanic 5% African American
Other clinical characteristics:	≥ 1 previous attempt: SBT=53 (8%) vs SRT=44 (7%) Major depressive disorder: SBT=27 (4%) vs SRT=31 (5%) Disruptive behavior disorder: SBT=27 (4%) vs SRT=63 (10%) Alcohol use disorder: SBT=13 (2%) vs SRT=25 (4%) Cannabis use disorder: SBT=40 (6%) vs SRT=50 (8%) Number of diagnoses: None: SBT=53 (8%) vs SRT=25 (4%); 1: SBT=20 (3%) vs SRT=38 (6%); >2: SBT=27 (4%) vs SRT= 38 (6%)
Concomitant medications:	50% selective serotonin reuptake inhibitor (SSRI) alone 33% SSRI plus another medication 6% atypical antidepressant 11% mood stabilizer
Outcome assessment:	Outcome measures were administered 3 months (end of active treatment) and 6 months (end of maintenance)
Results:	N=31 Reattempts at 6 months: SBT=26.7% (4/15) vs SRT=12.5% (2/16); χ^2=1.00 The difference in rates of suicide reattempts among those taking (n = 6/6) versus not taking (n = 0/25) medication was statistically significant: χ^2=7.95, $P < .05$
Author, Year (Country):	Green 2011[44] (UK)
Population:	Adolescents aged 12-17 years with at least 2 past episodes of self-harm within the previous 12 months.
Therapy 1:	Developmental group psychotherapy: manual-based treatment designed for self-harming adolescents. Integrated techniques including CBT, DBT, and group psychotherapy. Adolescents learned strategies to deal with difficulties using group based techniques such as role play.
Therapy 2:	Local child and adolescent mental health services teams provided standard routine care according to their clinical judgment. Centers excluded any group intervention from routine care during the trial.
Medication regimen:	None.
Setting:	Child and adolescent mental health service teams in the northwest of England, who served substantial geographical areas.
Therapist Duration:	Therapists had a minimum of 3 years of relevant post-qualifying experience; had initial training in fidelity to the model and subsequent regular supervision.
Treatment Duration:	Rolling entry; adolescents started attending as soon as their initial assessment and randomization were completed and attendance continued until the young person felt ready to leave. Mean number of group sessions attended was 102 (SD 10.1). Minimum per protocol adherence was 4 sessions per site per year.
N:	366 (183 group therapy, 183 usual care)
Mean age, % female, race (variance):	38% age 12 to 14 years at entry, 62% 15 to 17 years (mean ages not reported) 89% female 7% black and ethnic minority

Other clinical characteristics:	69% high psychosocial risk; 62% depressive disorder; 33% behavioral disorder
Concomitant medications:	Not reported
Outcome assessment:	Primary outcome was the frequency of episodes of self-harm (includes non-suicidal self-harm). Face-to-face interview, structured interviewing techniques, additional monthly telephone interview with patient and family.
Results:	3 episodes of self-harm resulting in severe physical injury (2 usual care, 1 group therapy). No suicides or other deaths.

Author, Year (Country):	Hatcher 2011[36] (New Zealand)
Population:	Patients over age 16 who presented to the hospital after self-harm between September 2005 and June 2008. Self-harm included: "intentional self-poisoning or self-injury, irrespective of motivation. Self-poisoning included the intentional ingestion of more than the prescribed amount of any drug, whether or not there was evidence that the act was intended to result in death. This also included poisoning with non-ingestible substances (for example pesticides or carpet cleaner), overdoses of 'recreational' drugs and severe alcohol intoxication where the clinical staff considered such cases to be an act of self-harm. Self-injury was defined as any injury that had been intentionally self-inflicted." Patients receiving DBT or other "management plan which precluded having a short-term therapy" were excluded from the study.
Intervention 1:	Treatment as usual (TAU): Varied and may involve referral to multidisciplinary teams for psychiatric or psychological intervention, referral to mental health crisis teams, recommendations for engagement with alcohol and drug treatment centers or other health and non-health services.
Intervention 2:	Problem-solving therapy plus treatment as usual (PST+TAU): Up to 9 hour-long sessions lasting up to 3 months. Conducted with individual patients in outpatient clinics. Steps included problem orientation, problem listing and definition, brainstorming, devising an action plan and reviewing the plan. Engaged people by getting them to tell the story of their attempt and understanding the motivation behind it. Conducted regular risk assessments and in the final sessions asked participants to apply their new skills to the circumstances around their original self-harm attempt.
Setting:	4 District Health Boards (hospitals providing healthcare to about a third of the New Zealand population).
N:	1094; PST+TAU=522, TAU=572
Mean age, % female, race (variance):	Age, years (SD): PST+TAU=33.2 (12.5) vs TAU=34.2 (13.2) % female: PST+TAU=68% vs TAU=69% Ethnicity (%): PST+TAU vs TAU: NZ European 62% vs 60%, Maori 14% vs 17%, Pacific Island 7% vs 5%, Asian 2% vs 4%, Other 15% vs 13%
Outcome assessment:	Primary outcome was presentation to hospital with self-harm in the year after the index attempt. Obtained from the New Zealand Health Information Service details of hospital contacts throughout New Zealand in the year after the index attempt. Data obtained from the National Minimum Dataset kept by the New Zealand health information service, which contains routinely collected information on all public and private hospital discharges in New Zealand.
Results:	Consenting Patients *Participants re-presenting to hospital for self-harm; PST+TAU vs TAU:* All index episodes (N=253 vs 299): 14.2% vs 17.1%; RR=0.17 (95% CI -0.24 to 0.44); P=0.43 Index episode is first self-harm episode (N=137 vs 169): 13.9% vs 8.9%; RR=-0.56 (95% CI -1.96 to 0.18); P=0.23 Index episode is repeat episode (N=116 vs 130): 14.7% vs 27.7%; RR=0.47 (95% CI 0.11 to 0.69); P=0.02; NNT=8 *Participants with self-reported self-harm; PST+TAU vs TAU:* All index episodes (N=186 vs 226): 27.4% vs 32.7%; RR=0.16 (95% CI -0.13 to 0.38); P=0.29 Index episode is first self-harm episode (N=98 vs 122): 25.5% vs 20.5%; RR= -0.25 (95% CI -1.03 to 0.24); P=0.47 Index episode is repeat episode (N=88 vs 104): 29.5% vs 47.1%; RR=0.37 (95% CI 0.08 to 0.57); P=0.02; NNT=6 *Time to re-presentation to hospital, days : median; PST+TAU vs TAU:* All index episodes: 56 vs 83; HR=0.81 (95% CI 0.53 to 1.25); P=0.92 Index episode is first self-harm episode: 62 vs 75; HR=1.62 (95% CI 0.82 to 3.18); P=0.16 Index episode is repeat episode: 45 vs 104; HR=0.47 (95% CI 0.26 to 0.85); P=0.01 All Patients *Participants re-presenting to hospital for self-harm; PST+TAU vs TAU:* All index episodes (N=522 vs 572): 13.4% vs 14.1%; RR=0.05 (95% CI -0.28 to 0.30); P=0.79 Index episode is first self-harm episode (N=314 vs 360): 13.4% vs 9.4%; RR=-0.42 (95% CI -1.17 to 0.08); P=0.37 Index episode is repeat episode (N=208 vs 212): 13.5% vs 22.1%; RR=0.39 (95% CI 0.07 to 0.60); P=0.03; NNT=12 *Time to re-presentation to hospital, days : median; PST+TAU vs TAU:* All index episodes: 74 vs 75; HR=0.98 (95% CI 0.71 to 1.36); P=0.92 Index episode is first self-harm episode: 74 vs 61; HR=1.55 (95% CI 0.98 to 2.48); P=0.06 Index episode is repeat episode: 80 vs 114; HR=0.58 (95% CI 0.36 to 0.94); P=0.03

Author, Year (Country):	Hazell 2009[49] (Australia)
Population:	Adolescents aged between 12 and 16 years, who had been referred to a child and adolescent mental health service in Australian sites at Newcastle, Brisbane North, or Logan, and reported at least 2 episodes of self-harm in the past year, 1 of which had occurred in the past 3 months
Therapy 1:	Group Therapy (GT): Developed by Wood et al. (2001) and administered as described in treatment manual (Wood 2001). One-hour group sessions conducted weekly. Initial 6 sessions focused on relationships, school and peer relationships, family problems, anger management, depression and self-harm, and hopelessness and feelings about the future. After completion of the initial 6 sessions, adolescents could transition to a longer term group for up to 12 months.
Therapy 2:	Routine Care (RC): Generally consisted of individual counseling (using a variety of therapeutic approaches), family sessions, medication assessment and review, and other care coordination activities
Medication regimen:	Details not reported
Setting:	Community-based adolescent mental health service
Therapist characteristics:	GT: Delivered by 2 clinicians from each participating community-based adolescent mental health service, who were qualified psychologists, clinical psychologists, social workers, or nurses and were supervised by chief investigators

RC: Also provided by community-based adolescent mental health services, but monitored via a self-report resource use surveys and the collection of information from electronic health records. |
| Treatment duration: | Up to 12 months |
| N: | 72 |
| Mean age, % female, race (variance): | Mean age, years (SD): GT=14.57 (1.07) vs RC=14.41 (1.19)
% Female: GT=91% vs RC=89%
Race not reported |
| Other clinical characteristics: | % Patients with:
At least 1 incident of medication overdose: GT=71% vs RC=43%
At least 1 incident of deliberate self-cutting: GT=100% vs RC=97%
Medically serious self-harm: GT=9% vs RC=5%
Lifetime probable or definite sexual abuse: GT=31% vs RC=32%
Alcohol problems: GT=6% vs RC=3%
Substance misuse: GT=0 vs RC=0
Depression: GT=49% vs RC=65%
Conduct/oppositional defiant disorder: GT=6% vs RC=8% |
| Concomitant medications: | Not reported |
| Outcome assessment: | Primary outcome measure was repetition of self-harm, defined as any intentional self-inflicted injury (including poisoning) irrespective of the apparent purpose of the behavior, based on an interview-based assessment of suicide behavior (Kerfoot 1992, Linehan 1999). |
| Results: | Repetition of Deliberate Self-Harm by 6 months: GT = 88% (30/34); RC = 68% (23/34); p = 0.04
Repetition of Deliberate Self-Harm in interval of 6 to 12 months: GT = 88% (30/34); RC = 71% (24/34); p = 0.07 |

Author, Year (Country):	Linehan 2006[38] (US)
Population:	Women between the ages of 18 and 45 years who met criteria for borderline personality disorder and for current and past suicidal behavior as defined by at least 2 suicide attempts or self-injuries n the past 5 years, with at least 1 in the past 8 weeks.
Therapy 1:	DBT: A cognitive behavioral treatment program developed to treat suicidal clients meeting criteria for BPD (Linehan 1993, Linehan 1993) that directly targets: 1) suicidal behavior, 2) behaviors that interfere with treatment delivery, and 3) other dangerous, severe, or destabilizing behaviors. Standard DBT addresses the following 5 functions: 1) increasing behavioral capabilities, 2) improving motivation for skillful behavior (through contingency management and reduction of interfering emotions and cognitions), 3) assuring generalization of gains to the natural environment, 4) structuring the treatment environment so that it reinforces functional rather than dysfunctional behaviors, and 5) enhancing therapist capabilities and motivation to treat patients effectively. These functions are divided among the following 4 modes of service delivery: 1) weekly individual psychotherapy (1 h/wk), 2) group skills training (2½ h/wk), 3) telephone consultation (as needed within the therapist's limits to ensure generalization), and (4) weekly therapist consultation team meetings (to enhance therapist motivation and skills and to provide therapy for the therapists).
Therapy 2:	Community Treatment By Experts (CTBE): This condition was developed specifically for this study to control for factors previously uncontrolled for in DBT studies. Similar to a TAU (treatment as usual) condition, the treatment provided was uncontrolled by the research team. Therapists were asked to provide the type and dose of therapy that they believed was most suited to the patient, with a minimum of 1 scheduled individual session per week. Ancillary treatment could be prescribed as needed. CTBE differs from TAU conditions in that characteristics of CTBE therapists are controlled by the study via selection of therapists and supervisory arrangements. CTBE therapists included heads of inpatient psychiatric units and clinical directors of mental health agencies.

Medication regimen:	Not reported
Setting:	Not reported
Therapist characteristics:	41 therapists (16 DBT and 25 CTBE therapists). Doctoral degree: DBT=75% vs CTBE=56% > 10 years' clinical experience since terminal degree: DBT=25% vs CTBE=56% Male: DBT=31.3% vs CTBE=36% Mean number of study clients: DBT=3.6 (2.9) vs CTBE=2.5 (1.7) Subjects in group consultation: DBT=100% vs 57.1%
Treatment duration:	1 year
N:	111: DBT=60 vs CTBE=51
Mean age, % female, race (variance):	Mean age, years (SD): 29.3 (7.5) 100% women White: 87% African American: 4% Native American: 2% Native American or Alaskan Native: 1% Other Race: 5%
Other clinical characteristics:	Current psychiatric diagnoses meeting *DSM-IV* criteria: Major depressive disorder=72.3%, Panic Disorder=40.6%, Post-Traumatic Stress Disorder=49.5%, Any Anxiety Disorder=78.2%, Any Substance Use Disorder=29.7%, Any Eating Disorder=23.8% Lifetime psychiatric diagnoses meeting *DSM-IV* criteria: Major depressive disorder=96%, Panic Disorder=51.5%, Post-Traumatic Stress Disorder=55.4%, Any Anxiety Disorder=87.1%, Any Substance Use Disorder=73.3%, Any Eating Disorder=39.6% Axis II: Cluster A=3.0%, Cluster B other than borderline personality disorder=10.9%, Cluster C=25.7%, Paranoid=3.0, Schizotypal=0.0, Antisocial=10.9%, Histrionic=2.0%, Narcissistic=0.0%, Avoidant=20.8%, Dependent=5.9%, Obsessive Compulsive=7.9%, Psychiatric Disorder Not Otherwise Specified=89.1% Median suicide attempts (interquartile range): 1.0 (0.5-4.0) Median nonsuicidal self-injury (interquartile range): 10.0 (2.0 to 47.0)
Concomitant medications:	Proportion of subjects taking any psychotropic medications (Estimated from Figure 2): 12 months: DBT=47% vs CTBE=69% 24 months: DBT=54% vs CTBE=63%
Outcome assessment:	The Suicide Attempt Self-Injury Interview (Seligman 2006) measured the topography, suicide intent, and medical severity of each suicide attempt and nonsuicidal self-injury. Assessments completed at 4-month intervals during the 12-month treatment and 12 months of post-treatment follow-up periods by blinded, independent clinical assessors with master's or doctoral degrees.
Results:	Median suicides (interquartile range): DBT=0 (0 to 0) vs CTBE=0 (0 to 1) Suicide attempts: DBT=23.1% vs CTBE=46%, *P*=0.01, HR=2.66 (95% CI not reported; *P*=0.005), NNT=4.24 (95% CI, 2.40 to 18.07) Nonambivalent suicide attempts: DBT=5.8% vs CTBE=13.3%, *P*=0.18, NNT=13.3 (95% CI, 5.28 to 25.41) Suicide attempts per period: Significantly fewer in the DBT group across the 2 years when controlling for number of suicide attempts during the pretreatment year (F1,94=3.20, *P*=.04, MMANOVA). Mean proportions of suicide attempters per period: DBT=6.2% (95% CI, 3.1% to 11.7%) vs CTBE=12.2% (95% CI, 7.1% to 20.3%)

Author, Year (Country):	**McMain 2009[42] (Canada)**
Population:	Patients who met DSM-IV criteria for borderline personality disorder (BPD), were 18–60 years of age, and had at least two episodes of suicidal or nonsuicidal self-injurious episodes in the past 5 years, at least one of which was in the 3 months preceding enrollment

Therapy 1:	DBT: A cognitive behavioral treatment program developed by Linehan (Linehan 1993, Linehan 1993), which includes the following components: *Theoretical basis*: Learning theory, Zen philosophy, and dialectical philosophy. Pervasive emotion dysregulation is the primary deficit in borderline personality disorder. *Treatment structure*: Multimodal: Individual sessions (1 hour weekly); skills group (2 hours weekly); phone coaching (2 hours weekly); consultation team for therapists mandated (2 hrs weekly); organized according to a hierarchy of targets: suicidal, treatment-interfering, and quality-of-life-interfering behaviors; explicit focus on self-harm and suicidal behavior *Primary strategies*: Psychoeducation about BPD, helping relationship, here-and-now focus, validation and empathy, emotion focus, dialectical strategies, irreverent and reciprocal communication style, formal skills training, behavioral strategies (e.g., exposure, contingency management, diary cards, behavioral aspects) *Crisis management protocols*: Bias toward managing crises on an outpatient basis; phone coaching to assist in managing crises
Therapy 2:	General Psychiatric Management. (GPM): Based on the APA Practice Guideline for the Treatment of Patients With Borderline Personality Disorder and included the following components: *Theoretical basis*: Psychodynamic approach drawn from Gunderson 2001; emphasized the relational aspects and early attachment relationships. Disturbed attachment relationships related to emotion dysregulation as a primary deficit. *Treatment structure*: One mode: Individual sessions (1 hour weekly) including medication management based on structured drug algorithm; therapist supervision meeting mandated (90 minutes weekly); patient preference is given priority—no hierarchy of targets; focus is expanded away from self-harm and suicidal behaviors. *Primary strategies*: Psychoeducation about BPD, helping relationship, here-and-now focus, validation and empathy, emotion focus, active attention to signs of negative transference. *Crisis management protocols*: Hospitalization if indicated.
Medication regimen:	DBT: Patients encouraged to rely on skills over pills where appropriate (e.g., anxiolytics). Tapering from medications was a treatment goal. Psychopharmacologic intervention was uncontrolled GPM: Patients were encouraged to use medications concurrently. Two medication algorithms, one related to mood lability and one related to impulsive-aggressiveness, were prioritized as symptom targets. Medication intervention was delivered according to the predominant symptom pattern.
Setting:	Treatments conducted at separate University of Toronto teaching hospitals within the same health care system. DBT was conducted at the Centre for Addiction and Mental Health and GPM at St. Michael's Hospital.
Therapist characteristics:	Treatments were delivered by 25 therapists, all with a minimum of 1 year of experience treatment borderline patients. Therapists included 11 psychiatrists (three and eight providing DBT and general psychiatric management, respectively), five Ph.D.-level psychologists (four and one, respectively), six master's-level clinicians (five and one, respectively), and three nurses (one and two, respectively). There were no between-group differences in the proportion of clinicians with doctoral-level degrees (M.D. and Ph.D.) versus other degrees, but there were significantly more physicians in the general psychiatric management condition (χ^2=4.8, df=1, p=0.028).
Treatment duration:	12 months
N:	180: DBT=90 vs GPM=90
Mean age, % female, race (variance):	Mean age, years (SD): 30.4 (9.9) 86.1% female Race not reported
Other clinical characteristics:	Lifetime DSM-IV axis I disorders, % patients: Major depressive disorder=80.0%, Panic disorder=31.7%, Post-Traumatic Stress Disorder=47.2%, any Anxiety Disorder=76.1%, any Substance Use Disorder=58.9%, any Eating Disorder=30.6% Current DSM-IV axis I and II diagnoses: Major depressive disorder=48.9%, Panic disorder=21.7%, Post-Traumatic Stress Disorder=37.4%, any Anxiety Disorder=75%, any Substance Use Disorder=9.4%, any Eating Disorder=13.3%, Axis II cluster A disorders=7.8%, Axis II cluster B diagnosis (excluding BPD)=17.8%, Axis II cluster C disorders=40.6% Mean lifetime suicide attempts (SD): 24.7 (88.3)
Concomitant medications:	Not reported.
Outcome assessment:	The primary outcome measures were frequency and severity of suicidal and nonsuicidal self-injurious behavior episodes, as assessed every 4 months by the Suicide Attempt Self-Injury Interview (M.M. Linehan et al., unpublished 1983 manuscript).
Results:	Deaths by suicide: None Mean number of suicidal and self-injurious episodes (SD): OR 0.92 (*P*=0.76) 4 months: DBT=10.60 (20.96) vs GPM=14.02 (43.87) 8 months: DBT=8.94 (19.07) vs GPM=11.44 (37.59) 12 months: DBT=4.29 (9.32) vs GPM=12.87 (51.45)

Author, Year (Country):	Stewart 2009[50] (Australia)
Population:	People aged 18 years or older receiving inpatient treatment for a suicide attempt.
Therapy 1:	CBT: based on a combination of Beck's CBT and Albert Ellis's theory of rational emotive therapy. Individual weekly sessions.
Therapy 2:	Problem-Solving Therapy (PST): based on the 6-step D'Zurilla and Goldfried model. Individual weekly sessions.
Medication regimen:	None
Setting:	2 hospitals in Australia
Therapist characteristics:	Treatments administered by the researcher (not described)
Treatment duration:	Sessions were one hour, with PST completed over 4 sessions and CBT over approximately 7 sessions.
N:	Unclear: states number of participants was 32, but also reports that 11 patients completed CBT, 12 PST, and 9 treatment as usual
Mean age, % female, race (variance):	Age range 20-58 years (mean not reported) 53% female Race not reported
Other clinical characteristics:	None reported.
Concomitant medications:	None reported.
Outcome assessment:	Four tests of psychological functioning, and repeated attempt data from hospital chart audits that recorded re-presentation to the hospital for suicide attempts. Measures administered when participants were initially screened, directly following treatment (for PST and CBT groups) and at 2-month follow-up (for the treatment as usual group).
Results:	Average number of suicide attempts: CBT: 0.22 (SD=0.64) PST: 0.33 (SD=0.63) TAU: 0.22 (SD=0.50) No significant differences found for repetition of suicide attempts when PST group was compared to TAU (U=35, ns, r=0.13) and when CBT was compared to TAU (U=25, ns, r=0.32)

Author, Year (Country):	Tarrier 2006[51] (UK)
Population:	DSM-4 criteria for schizophrenia, schizophreniform disorder, schizoaffective disorder, delusional disorder or psychosis not otherwise specified; either first or second admission to inpatient or daypatient unit for treatment of psychosis; positive psychotic symptoms for 4 weeks or more.
Therapy 1:	CBT: Manual-based and supervised. Addressed delusions and hallucinations, generating alternative hypotheses for abnormal beliefs and hallucinations, identifying precipitating and alleviating factors and reducing associated distress, and teaching coping strategies.
Therapy 2:	Supportive counseling (SC). Delivered in the same 5-week format with 3 boosters, with the aim of matching the duration of total therapist contact time to that in the CBT arm. SC was manual based and supervised; the same 5 therapists administered both interventions.
Therapy 2:	Treatment as usual
Medication regimen:	None as part of the intervention
Setting:	11 mental health units serving 3 geographically defined catchment areas.
Therapist characteristics:	5 therapists trained in CBT for psychosis; 3 were clinical psychologists and 2 nurse therapists
Treatment duration:	Aimed for 15-20 hours treatment envelope within a 5-week post-admission period, plus booster sessions at a further 2 weeks, and 1, 2, and 3 months.
N:	278; unclear how many in each group
Mean age, % female, race (variance):	Not reported by treatment group; reported by low self-harm score (N=242) and high self-harm score (N=36): Mean age, years (SD): 29.7 (10.6) and 28.6 (6.4) % female: 30.6% Ethnic minority (not specified): 12.2%
Other clinical characteristics:	35% detained under MHA 35% no substance misuse; 13.7% daily substance misuse
Concomitant medications:	Chlorpromazine equivalents: mean (SD) Low self-harm score=489.3 (374.4) mg High self-harm score=537.2 (460.2) mg

Outcome assessment:	Deaths for any reason identified from hospital and psychiatric notes. Suicides and possible suicides (where the death might have been intentional or accidental and the coroner ruled the death as accidental) were identified. Suicide ideation and behavior (combined) assessed by the non-accidental self injury scale of the HoNOS (Health of the Nation Outcome Scales). Serious risk (score of 4) indicates suicidal attempts or deliberate self-harm. Assessed at 6 weeks, 3 months, and 18 months.
Results:	Over 18 months, there were 3 definite suicides (1.2%), 2 in the supportive counseling group and 1 in CBT group. Two further deaths classified as accidental by the coroner (1 traffic accident, 1 fall from window, 1 in supportive counseling group, 1 in CBT group). 2 deaths by natural causes. Numbers too small for meaningful statistical analysis. On the HoNOS, there were no significant differences between the 3 treatment groups at any time point. Psychological treatment did not significantly reduce or worsen suicidal behavior compared to treatment as usual. There was a marked reduction in suicidal behavior after admission that would mask any potential treatment effect.
Author, Year (Country):	**Unutzer 2006[52] (US)**
Population:	Aged 60 and older, met criteria for current major depression, dysthymia, or both, and planned to use one of the participating primary care clinics over the following year.
Intervention 1:	IMPACT intervention: 1-year collaborative care program that included a Depression Care manager (DCM, nurses and psychologists). DCMs completed an initial assessment visit and provided education about treatment options, including antidepressant medications and psychotherapy. All patients were encouraged to engage in behavioral activation and offered a choice of treatment with antidepressant medications, or Problem Solving Treatment in Primary Care, a brief behavioral intervention lasting between 4 and 8 sessions that non-mental health providers provide. DCMs received weekly supervision from a PCP and a psychiatrist to monitor progress and adjust treatment plans according to a stepped-care treatment algorithm. The DCM followed patients in person or by telephone approximately every 2 weeks during acute-phase treatment and monthly during the continuation phase.
Intervention 2:	Usual care: patients and their PCPs were told that patients met research diagnostic criteria for major depression or dysthymia. Patients could receive all treatments available, including antidepressant medications or counseling by their PCPs, as well as referral to specialty mental health care.
Setting:	18 primary care clinics affiliated with healthcare organizations in 5 states (Indiana, Texas, North Carolina, California, Washington).
N:	1801; IMPACT=906, Usual care=895
Mean age, % female, race (variance):	IMPACT vs Usual care Age, years (SD): 71.01 (7.35) vs 71.35 (7.6) % female: 64.1% vs 65.6% White: 78.2% vs 75.9% African American: 12.6% vs 12.1% Latino: 6.2% vs 9.1% Other race/ethnicity: 3.0% vs 2.9%
Outcome assessment:	Primary outcome was suicidal ideation. No information on how deaths were ascertained.
Results:	117 participants died before the 24-month follow-up; 61 of them (52%) were in the intervention group. To the authors' knowledge, there were no suicides in either group during the 2-year study period.
Comments	A suicide prevention protocol was in place for both groups: Patients who endorsed thoughts of suicide were asked if they thought they might act on these feelings; if they answered yes or refused to answer, the interviewer encouraged the patient to discuss these thoughts with a professional and offered telephone numbers including a 24-hour emergency contact number and a suicide hotline. The protocol was activated 135 times for 108 study patients (89 times usual care vs 46 times intervention). Of the patients who triggered the risk-reduction protocol, 7.7% were in the usual care group and 4.3% in the intervention group (P<0.01)
Author, Year (Country):	**Winter 2007[43] (UK)**
Population:	People attending two Accident and Emergency departments following episodes of self-harm.
Therapy 1:	Personal construct psychotherapy. Techniques were selected on the basis of their likely impact on the client's construing. Therapeutic techniques appropriate to particular personal construct formulations of the client's self-harm were set out in a brief manual.
Therapy 2:	Normal clinical practice: Assessment by, and possible follow-up appointments with, a mental health team. In one of the Accident and Emergency departments, a psychiatric crisis team visited the client while in the department; in the other, an appointment was made for him/her to attend a psychiatric outpatient clinic.
Medication regimen:	None as part of the intervention
Setting:	Accident and Emergency departments serving a North London Borough
Therapist characteristics:	Clinical psychologist, supervised by an experienced personal construct psychotherapist.
Treatment duration:	Six-session contract, commencing soon after the self-harm, which could be renewed if agreed by therapist and client. Number of sessions ranged from 2 to 22 (mean 10.38 sessions)
N:	40: 24 intervention, 40 control

Mean age, % female, race (variance):	Intervention vs control. Mean age, years (SD)= 33.88 (7.66) vs 35.83 (10.43) % female=42% vs 60% White ethnic group=100%
Other clinical characteristics:	No additional relevant information
Concomitant medications:	Not reported
Outcome assessment:	Primary outcomes were measure of suicidal ideation and depression. For assessment of self-harm, records from the Accident and Emergency departments involved in the study were monitored for repeat episodes of self-harm in the 3 years following their initial presentation.
Results:	Repetition of deliberate self-harm, intervention vs control At 1 year: 17% vs 36% (P=0.12) At 3 years: 35% vs 53% (P=0.18) At 5 years: 39% vs 58% (P=0.15) No repetition within 5 years: 61% vs 42% (P not reported) 3 of the episodes eventuated in successful suicide (1 intervention, 2 control)

APPENDIX R. RISK OF BIAS RATINGS FOR PRIMARY STUDIES RELATED TO PSYCHOTHERAPY

Author Year	Sequence Generation — Was it adequate? Yes/No/Unclear; Describe method	Allocation concealment — Was it adequate? Yes/No/Unclear; Describe method	Blinding of participants, personnel, and outcome assessors — Describe all measures used, if any, to blind study participants and personnel from knowledge of which intervention participant received. Provide any information relating to whether intended blinding was effective. Was knowledge of allocated intervention adequately prevented during study? Yes/No/Unclear	Incomplete outcome data — Describe completeness of outcome data for each main outcome, including attrition and exclusions from the analysis. State whether attrition and exclusions were reported, numbers in each intervention group (compared with total randomized participants), reasons for attrition/exclusions where reported, and any re-inclusions in analyses performed by review authors. Were incomplete outcome data adequately addressed? Yes/No/Unclear	Selective outcome reporting — State how possibility of selective outcome reporting was examined by review authors, and what was found. Are reports of study free of suggestion of selective outcome reporting? Yes/No/Unclear	Other sources of bias — State any important concerns about bias not addressed in other domains in tool. If particular questions/entries were pre-specified in review's protocol, responses should be provided for each question/entry. Was study apparently free of other problems that could put it at high risk of bias? Yes/No/Unclear	OVERALL risk of bias for study as a whole — Low/Unclear/High
Bateman 2008[117]	Unclear. No information provided other than stating that patients were randomized following the initial assessment.	Unclear. No information provided.	No. Not described, does not appear to be blinded.	No. Attritions and exclusions adequately documented; subject flowchart included in article. Analyzed 36/44 (82%). 3 patients in control group crossed over to treatment group after suicide attempts; 3 patients dropped out of treatment. These were not included in analysis. At 8-year follow-up: results on 41 patients.	Yes. Methods published prior to results.	No. Reports baseline characteristics only on those included in analysis (36 of 44 randomized).	High
Bateman 2009[37]	Yes. "Randomization followed consent, enrollment, and baseline assessment... Treatment allocation was made offsite via telephone randomization using a stochastic minimization program (MINIM) balancing for age, gender, and presence of antisocial personality disorder."	Yes. "Treatment allocation was made offsite via telephone randomization."	Assessors: Yes; Participants: No. "A study psychiatrist informed participants of their assignment." "Assessors were blind to treatment group." The study was designed to compare to a well-matched alternative treatment provided in similar contexts by similarly trained therapists and, therefore, even though patients may have been aware of the type of treatment they were receiving, both treatments were likely perceived as effective treatment methods.	Yes. Attritions and exclusions adequately documented; subject flowchart included in article. 134/134 analyzed.	Yes. No omissions of any expected suicide-related outcomes; authors state that primary outcomes were declared prior to beginning the study.	Unclear. Those who declined participation were more likely to have history of alcohol abuse (N=12); reported rape at baseline was more common in MBT group. No information is provided re: possible nesting (e.g., therapist effects). Unclear- may have been other unmeasured differences at baseline.	Unclear

Author Year	Sequence Generation		Allocation concealment		Blinding of participants, personnel, and outcome assessors		Incomplete outcome data		Selective outcome reporting		Other sources of bias		OVERALL risk of bias for study as a whole
	Was it adequate? Yes/No/ Unclear	Describe method	Was it adequate? Yes/No/ Unclear	Describe method	Describe all measures used, if any, to blind study participants and personnel from knowledge of which intervention participant received. Provide any information relating to whether intended blinding was effective.	Was knowledge of allocated intervention adequately prevented during study? Yes/No/ Unclear	Describe completeness of outcome data for each main outcome, including attrition and exclusions from the analysis. State whether attrition and exclusions were reported, numbers in each intervention group (compared with total randomized participants), reasons for attrition/ exclusions where reported, and any re-inclusions in analyses performed by review authors.	Were incomplete outcome data adequately addressed? Yes/No/ Unclear	State how possibility of selective outcome reporting was examined by review authors, and what was found.	Are reports of study free of suggestion of selective outcome reporting? Yes/No/ Unclear	State any important concerns about bias not addressed in other domains in tool. If particular questions/ entries were pre-specified in review's protocol, responses should be provided for each question/ entry.	Was study apparently free of other problems that could put it at high risk of bias? Yes/No/ Unclear	Low/ Unclear/ High
Blum 2008[39]	Yes	Coin toss.	Yes	Coin toss occurred following inclusion in study; therefore, allocation was unknown when determining treatment condition.	No information provided. Because the comparison group (TAU) could likely be identified as such by participants, lack of participant blinding could introduce significant bias.	Unclear	Missing data, attritions, and exclusions adequately reported. Those with at least one post-baseline assessment included in analysis: 124/165.	No	No omissions of any expected suicide-related outcomes.	Yes	Reports baseline characteristics on 124/165 randomized (those who received the intervention); avoidant personality disorder more frequent in treatment as usual alone group (P=0.016). Because it is unclear whether or not the two treatment therapists conducted the groups together or separately, these nesting effects may not have been adequately addressed.	No	High
Comtois 2011[47]	Yes	"Minimization algorithm matching for gender, history of suicide attempt, pre-existing use of psychotropic medications, and history of substance abuse."	Unclear	No information provided.	"Primary outcome variables… were assessed by a licensed clinician blind to treatment condition." No information on provider or patient blinding.	Yes for assessors, unclear for participants.	Attritions and exclusions documented; however, 12/16 (75%) of treatment and 10/16 (62.5%) of control participants did not complete study.	No	No omissions of any expected suicide-related outcomes.	Yes	Two "severe and complex" patients removed from treatment condition; one control participant removed due to being court-ordered into an alternative treatment. No demographic or outcome data reported for completers vs. non-completers.	Yes	High

Author Year	Sequence Generation		Allocation concealment		Blinding of participants, personnel, and outcome assessors		Incomplete outcome data		Selective outcome reporting		Other sources of bias		OVERALL risk of bias for study as a whole
	Describe method	Was it adequate? Yes/No/Unclear	Describe method	Was it adequate? Yes/No/Unclear	Describe all measures used, if any, to blind study participants and personnel from knowledge of which intervention participant received. Provide any information relating to whether intended blinding was effective.	Was knowledge of allocated intervention adequately prevented during study? Yes/No/Unclear	Describe completeness of outcome data for each main outcome, including attrition and exclusions from the analysis. State whether attrition and exclusions were reported, numbers in each intervention group (compared with total randomized participants), reasons for attrition/exclusions where reported, and any re-inclusions in analyses performed by review authors.	Were incomplete outcome data adequately addressed? Yes/No/Unclear	State how possibility of selective outcome reporting was examined by review authors, and what was found.	Are reports of study free of suggestion of selective outcome reporting? Yes/No/Unclear	State any important concerns about bias not addressed in other domains in tool. If particular questions/entries were pre-specified in review's protocol, responses should be provided for each question/entry.	Was study apparently free of other problems that could put it at high risk of bias? Yes/No/Unclear	Low/ Unclear/ High
Davidson 2006[40]	Randomization schedules "generated by the study data center".	Yes	Blinded researcher contacted trial coordinator by phone to initiate a randomization.	Yes	Research assistants carried out all assessments and were blind to treatment group allocation; they requested that patients did not mention any details of any psychological treatment they were receiving.	Yes	Attritions and exclusions adequately documented. Follow-up data reported on 102/106 (96%).	Yes	Methods published prior to results.	Yes	The study appears to be free of other sources of bias.	Yes	Low
Diamond 2010[46]	Adaptive or "urn" randomization procedure, with four stratification variables: age, gender, past suicide attempt, and family conflict	Yes	Randomization described as "maintained by statistician", but no information about allocation	Unclear	Study participants, personnel and outcome assessors were all unblinded.	No	ITT; attrition reasonable overall (14%) and balanced between groups, but reasons not reported	Unclear	Protocol available at clinicaltrials. gov and primary outcomes are consistent. No omissions of any expected suicide-related outcomes.	Yes	The study appears to be free of other sources of bias.	Yes	Unclear
De Leo 2007[45]	Method not described ("randomization numbers")	Unclear	Sealed envelopes	Yes	Patients and case managers not blinded; no information on blinding of outcome assessors	No	High and differential attrition: 22/60 completed 12 months of treatment; 14/30 in intervention group vs 8/30 in treatment as usual group (47% vs 27%)	No	No indication of publication bias; outcomes described in methods are reported in results	Unclear	None noted	Yes	High

	Sequence Generation		Allocation concealment		Blinding of participants, personnel, and outcome assessors		Incomplete outcome data		Selective outcome reporting		Other sources of bias		OVERALL risk of bias for study as a whole
Author Year	Describe method	Was it adequate? Yes/No/ Unclear	Describe method	Was it adequate? Yes/No/ Unclear	Describe all measures used, if any, to blind study participants and personnel from knowledge of which intervention participant received. Provide any information relating to whether intended blinding was effective.	Was knowl-edge of allocated interven-tion ad-equately prevented during study? Yes/No/ Unclear	Describe completeness of outcome data for each main outcome, including attrition and exclusions from the analysis. State whether attrition and exclusions were reported, numbers in each intervention group (compared with total randomized participants), reasons for attrition/ exclusions where reported, and any re-inclusions in analyses performed by review authors.	Were in-complete outcome data ad-equately ad-dressed? Yes/No/ Unclear	State how possibility of selective outcome reporting was examined by review authors, and what was found.	Are reports of study free of sugges-tion of selective outcome report-ing? Yes/No/ Unclear	State any important concerns about bias not addressed in other domains in tool. If particular questions/ entries were pre-specified in review's protocol, responses should be provided for each question/ entry.	Was study appar-ently free of other problems that could put it at high risk of bias? Yes/No/ Unclear	Low/ Unclear/ High
Donaldson 2005[40]	No information provided other than stating that patients were randomized following the initial assessment.	Unclear	No information provided.	Unclear	The same 6 therapists administered two types of treatments and, therefore, were not blinded. No information on assessor blinding.	No	Demographic comparisons of completers and non-completers; ITT analysis. 31/39 (79%) randomized completed treatment and included in analysis.	No	No omissions of any expected suicide-related outcomes.	Yes	Baseline characteristics reported only for 31 who completed treatment; compared those who remained to those who dropped out and found no differences, but might have been differences between groups at baseline. The same therapists provided both treatments. No statistical techniques were used to account for nested data (e.g., therapist effects).	No	High
Green 2011[44]	Allocation was by minimization controlling for factors chosen as likely to predict treatment response	Unclear (sequence generation method not reported)	Randomization by remote telephone to trial center	Yes	Participants were not blinded (therapy study) Outcome assessors were blinded	Yes (for outcome assessors)	High and differential attrition: 37% in routine care group and 21% in therapy group did not receive intervention. But ITT analysis: 359/366 included in ITT analysis (98%); reasons for attrition reported adequately.	Yes	Results for stated primary outcomes are reported	Yes	None noted	Yes	Unclear
Hatcher 2011[36]	Computer-generated random numbers.	Yes	Independent statistician, sealed envelopes.	Yes	Patients blinded due to Zelen design; no therapist blinding for PST intervention and unclear for TAU providers; no information on blinding related to health record outcomes.	Yes for patients; unclear for providers; unclear for raters.	Significant loss to follow-up in consented patients, though 100% follow-up of hospital representation outcome because this was obtained for both consenting and non-consenting patients.	Yes	Outcomes and subgroup analyses determined *a priori*.	Yes	Patients receiving DBT were excluded from the study, and this could potentially result in a biased sample of patients.	Unclear	Low

106

	Sequence Generation		Allocation concealment		Blinding of participants, personnel, and outcome assessors		Incomplete outcome data		Selective outcome reporting		Other sources of bias		OVERALL risk of bias for study as a whole
	Describe method	Was it adequate? Yes/No/Unclear	Describe method	Was it adequate? Yes/No/Unclear	Describe all measures used, if any, to blind study participants and personnel from knowledge of which intervention participant received. Provide any information relating to whether intended blinding was effective.	Was knowledge of allocated intervention adequately prevented during study? Yes/No/Unclear	Describe completeness of outcome data for each main outcome, including attrition and exclusions from the analysis. State whether attrition and exclusions were reported, numbers in each intervention group (compared with total randomized participants), reasons for attrition/ exclusions where reported, and any re-inclusions in analyses performed by review authors.	Were incomplete outcome data adequately addressed? Yes/No/Unclear	State how possibility of selective outcome reporting was examined by review authors, and what was found.	Are reports of study free of suggestion of selective outcome reporting? Yes/No/Unclear	State any important concerns about bias not addressed in other domains in tool. If particular questions/ entries were pre-specified in review's protocol, responses should be provided for each question/ entry.	Was study apparently free of other problems that could put it at high risk of bias? Yes/No/Unclear	Low/Unclear/High
Author Year													
Hazell 2009[49]	No information provided other than stating that patients were randomized.	Unclear	Assigned by distant site coordinator	Yes	No patient and therapist blinding. Outcome assessor blinding attempted, but at end of follow-up, raters correctly identified the treatment allocation for 54% of participants: 65% in routine care group vs. 43% in experimental treatment group; p>0.06.	No for patient and therapist. Unclear for raters.	Data missing for 3% in experimental group and 8% in routine care group. Reasons not reported.	Yes	Prospectively-registered protocol not available. But, no omissions of any expected suicide-related outcomes	Yes	The study appears to be free of other sources of bias.	Yes	Unclear
Linehan, 2006[38]	"Using a computerized adaptive minimization randomization procedure, eligible subjects were matched to treatment condition on 5 primary diagnostic variables."	Yes	"The participant coordinator, who was not blinded to treatment condition, executed the randomization program and collected all the data related to treatment."	Unclear	"The participant coordinator, who was not blinded to treatment condition, executed the randomization program and collected all the data related to treatment." "Assessments were conducted by blinded independent clinical assessors." "Initial assessments were done before informing subjects of treatment assignment." Notably, the study was designed to compare to a well-matched alternative treatment provided in similar contexts by similarly trained therapists and, therefore, even though patients may have been aware of the type of treatment they were receiving, both treatments were likely perceived as effective treatment methods.	Assessors: yes; participants: no; providers: no.	"To assess the potential effect of missing data.... a pattern-mixture analysis was implemented using 2-tailed tests." Found no evidence that results were biased by these differences (data not reported). Attritions and exclusions clearly documented and accounted for in analyses; subject flowchart included in article.	Yes	No omissions of any expected suicide-related outcomes.	Yes	Differences in amount of therapy received in the different groups (DBT received more than CTBE due to weekly group sessions and greater treatment retention). Statistical techniques adequately accounted for nested data structures.	Unclear	Unclear

Author Year	Sequence Generation		Allocation concealment		Blinding of participants, personnel, and outcome assessors		Incomplete outcome data		Selective outcome reporting		Other sources of bias		OVERALL risk of bias for study as a whole
	Was it adequate? Yes/No/Unclear	Describe method	Was it adequate? Yes/No/Unclear	Describe method	Describe all measures used, if any, to blind study participants and personnel of which intervention participant received. Provide any information relating to whether intended blinding was effective.	Was knowledge of allocated intervention adequately prevented during study? Yes/No/Unclear	Describe completeness of outcome data for each main outcome, including attrition and exclusions from the analysis. State whether attrition and exclusions were reported, numbers in each intervention group (compared with total randomized participants), reasons for attrition/ exclusions where reported, and any re-inclusions in analyses performed by review authors.	Were incomplete outcome data adequately addressed? Yes/No/Unclear	State how possibility of selective outcome reporting was examined by review authors, and what was found.	Are reports of study free of suggestion of selective outcome reporting? Yes/No/Unclear	State any important concerns about bias not addressed in other domains in tool. If particular questions/ entries were pre-specified in review's protocol, responses should be provided for each question/ entry.	Was study apparently free of other problems that could put it at high risk of bias? Yes/No/Unclear	Low/ Unclear/ High
McMain 2009[42]	Unclear	Pre-generated random block sequence enclosed in envelopes. "Developed by a statistician," but unclear how.	Unclear	Scheme was held by statistician, who prepared 45 sealed envelopes, each containing the group allocations in random order for 4 participants; but no information about whether envelopes were sequentially numbered. Also concerned about potential clinical importance of ≥ 10% higher rates of lifetime anxiety and eating disorders, and current PTSD and substance use in DBT group.	Described as single blind. Explicit statements that assessors were blinded. When assessors were asked to guess treatment assignment, they were incorrect for 86% of cases, "suggesting blinding was largely maintained." Notably, the study was designed to compare to a well-matched alternative treatment provided in similar contexts by similarly trained therapists and, therefore, even though patients may have been aware of the type of treatment they were receiving, both treatments were likely perceived as effective treatment methods.	Assessors: yes; participants: no; providers: no.	ITT was conducted, but no information about imputation method. Attrition: 38% (DBT=39% vs. GPM=38%). Most common reasons for discontinuation of treatment were "individual sessions were not helpful (42%), scheduling problems (32%), transportation problems (32%), group sessions not helpful (29%), and that problems improved (24%)".	Unclear	No omissions of any expected suicide-related outcomes.	Yes	The study appears to be free of other sources of bias. No information is provided re: possible nested (e.g., therapist effects).	Yes	Unclear
Stewart 2009[90]	Unclear	Method not described	Unclear	Method not described	No information on blinding	Unclear	High and differential attrition: 34.4%, 37.5%, and 26.1% completed CBT, PST, and TAU interventions. Number included is given as 32. Number analyzed is not clear; one outlier was eliminated before data analysis.	No	No information to judge; "outcome measures included..."	Unclear	None noted	Yes	High

Author Year	Sequence Generation		Allocation concealment		Blinding of participants, personnel, and outcome assessors		Incomplete outcome data		Selective outcome reporting		Other sources of bias		OVERALL risk of bias for study as a whole
	Was it adequate? Yes/No/ Unclear	Describe method	Was it adequate? Yes/No/ Unclear	Describe method	Describe all measures used, if any, to blind study participants and personnel from knowledge of which intervention participant received. Provide any information relating to whether intended blinding was effective.	Was knowl-edge of allocated interven-tion ad-equately prevented during study? Yes/No/ Unclear	Describe completeness of outcome data for each main outcome, including attrition and exclusions from the analysis. State whether attrition and exclusions were reported, numbers in each intervention group (compared with total randomized participants), reasons for attrition/ exclusions where reported, and any re-inclusions in analyses performed by review authors.	Were in-complete outcome data ad-equately ad-dressed? Yes/No/ Unclear	State how possibility of selective outcome reporting was examined by review authors, and what was found.	Are reports of study free of sugges-tion of selective outcome report-ing? Yes/No/ Unclear	State any important concerns about bias not addressed in other domains in tool. If particular questions/ entries were pre-specified in review's protocol, responses should be provided for each question/ entry.	Was study appar-ently free of other problems that could put it at high risk of bias? Yes/No/ Unclear	Low/ Unclear/ High
Tarrier 2006[51]	Unclear	No information provided other than stating that patients were randomized.	Yes	"The interventions were carried out independently of assessors who were kept unaware of treatment allocation." Study personnel assigning treatment/ control condition were unaware of allocation.	The same 5 therapists administered 2 types of treatments and, therefore, were not blinded. Assessors were blinded to treatment allocation; deaths determined by review of hospital records.	Assessors: yes; participants: no; providers: no.	Attritions and exclusions adequately documented and subject flowchart included in article. For suicidal behavior, 71% follow-up at 18 months (218/278); for deaths, appears to be complete information.	No	No omissions of any expected suicide-related outcomes.	Yes	The same therapists provided both treat-ments. No statistical techniques were used to account for nested data (e.g., therapist or facility effects). In addition to suicides, 2 deaths were classified as accidental by the coroner and 2 deaths by natural causes (but possible to do calculations using this information).	No	High
Unutzer 2006[52]	Unclear	No information provided other than general statement of randomization.	Unclear	No information provided.	Telephone survey team blinded to intervention status (surveys measured suicidal ideation); for deaths, unclear if blinded.	Unclear	Unclear if missing data for deaths.	Unclear	No omissions of any expected suicide-related outcomes.	Yes	Primary outcome was suicidal thoughts; 117 patients died during follow-up: "to the authors' knowledge there were no suicides." No information on how this was determined or if data are complete.	No	Unclear
Winter 2007[43]	No	Not randomized: total randomization of the allocation to conditions was not possible... participants were allocated to the psychotherapy condition if there was a vacancy or to the normal clinical practice condition if not.	No	Not concealed.	Does not appear to be blinded (medical records were monitored for repeat episodes of self-harm).	No	Very high and differential attrition: 64 allocated, 45% control and 92% intervention completed post-treatment assessment; 28% and 54% completed 6-month assessment. However, information on repetition of self-harm behavior was traced in all participants over 3 years.	No	No omissions of any expected suicide-related outcomes.	Yes	Differences at baseline in 2 of 10 personal construct categories of self-harm.	No	High

APPENDIX S. STRENGTH OF EVIDENCE RATINGS FOR PRIMARY STUDIES RELATED TO PSYCHOTHERAPY[a]

Table 1. Attached-Based Family Therapy

| Number of studies; # of subjects | Domains pertaining to strength of evidence | | | | Magnitude of effect | Strength of evidence |
	Risk of bias (Design/ Risk of bias)	Consistency	Directness	Precision	Magnitude of effect	High, Moderate, Low, Insufficient
Attached-Based Family Therapy versus Enhanced Usual Care (Diamond 2010)[46]						
Low lethality suicide attempts						
1; 66	Medium (RCT/Unclear)	N/A	Indirect	Imprecise	ABFT = 11% (4/35); EUC = 22% (7/31); *p* not reported	Low

Table 2. Cognitive and Cognitive Behavioral Therapies (CBT)

| Number of studies; # of subjects | Domains pertaining to strength of evidence | | | | Magnitude of effect | Strength of evidence |
	Risk of bias (Design/ Risk of bias)	Consistency	Directness	Precision	Magnitude of effect	High, Moderate, Low, Insufficient
Cognitive Therapy for suicide attempters versus Usual Care (Brown 2005 as cited in Mann 2005)[10]						
Suicide re-attempt rate						
1; not reported	Medium (RCT/Unclear)	N/A	Indirect	N/A	"Halved event rate" reported in Mann 2005	Insufficient to Low
CBT for Cluster B Personality Disorders versus treatment as usual (Davidson 2010)[41]						
Number of subjects with suicidal acts from 0-6 years						
1; 106	Low (RCT/Low)	N/A	Indirect	Imprecise	aOR = 0.37 (95% CI, 0.10 to 1.38)	Low
Mean episodes of suicidal acts from 0-6 years						
1; 106	Low (RCT/Low)	N/A	Indirect	Imprecise	aMD (TAU-CBT) = 1.26 (95% CI, -0.06 to 2.58)	Low
CBT versus Supportive Counseling (Tarrier 2006)[51]						
Deaths by suicide after 18 months						
1; 278	High (RCT/High)	N/A	Indirect	Imprecise	CBT = 1; SC = 2; p not reported	Insufficient
CBT versus Problem Solving Therapy versus Usual Care (Stewart 2009)[50] Repeated in Problem Solving Therapy table below						
Average number of suicide attempts						
1; 32	High (RCT/High)	N/A	Indirect	Imprecise	CBT: 0.22 PST: 0.33 TAU: 0.22 No significant differences found for repetition of suicide attempts when PST group was compared to TAU	Insufficient

Table 3. Collaborative Assessment and Management of Suicidality (CAMS)

| Number of studies; # of subjects | Domains pertaining to strength of evidence | | | | Magnitude of effect | Strength of evidence |
	Risk of bias (Design/ Risk of bias)	Consistency	Directness	Precision	Magnitude of effect	High, Moderate, Low, Insufficient
CAMS versus E-CAU (Comtois 2011)[47]						
Mean number of suicide attempts and self-inflicted injuries at 12 months						
1; 32	High (RCT/High)	N/A	Indirect	Imprecise	Mean (SD): CAMS=1.2 (3.9) vs E-CAU=3.3 (7.6). P not reported.	Insufficient

Table 4. Dialectical Behavior Therapy (DBT)

| Number of studies; # of subjects | Domains pertaining to strength of evidence | | | | Magnitude of effect | Strength of evidence |
	Risk of bias (Design/ Risk of bias)	Consistency	Directness	Precision	Magnitude of effect	High, Moderate, Low, Insufficient
DBT versus Community Treatment By Experts (Linehan 2006)[38]						
Median suicides (interquartile range)						
1; 111	Medium (RCT/Unclear)	N/A	Indirect	Imprecise	DBT=0 (0 to 0) vs CTBE=0 (0 to 1)	Insufficient
Suicide attempts						
1; 111	Medium (RCT/Unclear)	N/A	Indirect	Imprecise	DBT=23.1% vs CTBE=46%, P=0.01, HR=2.66 (95% CI not reported; P=0.005), NNT=4.24 (95% CI, 2.40 to 18.07)	Low
DBT versus Standard Care (Hawton 2000 as cited in Mann 2005)[10]						
Unclear outcome reported in Mann 2005						
1 systematic review; not reported	Medium (SR/Unclear)	N/A	Indirect	N/A	Not reported	Insufficient to Low
DBT versus General Psychiatric Management (McMain 2009)[42]						
Deaths by suicide						
1; 180	Medium (RCT/Unclear)	N/A	Indirect	Imprecise	No events	Insufficient
Mean number of suicidal and self-injurious episodes at 12 months						
1; 180	Medium (RCT/Unclear)	N/A	Indirect	Imprecise	DBT=4.29 (9.32) vs GPM=12.87 (51.45); OR 0.92 (P=0.76)	Low

Table 5. Group Therapy

Number of studies; # of subjects	Domains pertaining to strength of evidence				Magnitude of effect	Strength of evidence
	Risk of bias (Design/ Risk of bias)	Consistency	Directness	Precision	Magnitude of effect	High, Moderate, Low, Insufficient
Group Therapy versus Routine Care (Hazell 2009)[49]						
Repetition of Deliberate Self-Harm by 6 months						
1; 72	Medium (RCT/Unclear)	N/A	Indirect	Imprecise	GT = 88% (30/34); RC = 68% (23/34); $p = 0.04$	Low
Repetition of Deliberate Self-Harm in interval of 6 to 12 months						
1; 72	Medium (RCT/Unclear)	N/A	Indirect	Imprecise	GT = 88% (30/34); RC = 71% (24/34); $p = 0.07$	Low
Group Therapy versus Routine Care (Green 2011)[44]						
Self-harm resulting in severe physical injury at 12 months						
1; 366	Medium (RCT/Unclear)	N/A	Indirect	Imprecise	Group therapy: 1/183 Usual care: 2/183 P not reported	Low
Suicide death at 12 months						
1; 366	Medium (RCT/Unclear)	N/A	Indirect	Imprecise	No events	Low

Table 6. IMPACT intervention

Number of studies; # of subjects	Domains pertaining to strength of evidence				Magnitude of effect	Strength of evidence
	Risk of bias (Design/ Risk of bias)	Consistency	Directness	Precision	Magnitude of effect	High, Moderate, Low, Insufficient
IMPACT intervention versus Usual Care (Unutzer 2006)[52]						
Deaths by suicide after 24 months						
1; 1801	Medium (RCT/Unclear)	N/A	Indirect	Imprecise	No events	Insufficient

Table 7. Intensive Care Plus Outreach

Number of studies; # of subjects	Domains pertaining to strength of evidence				Magnitude of effect	Strength of evidence
	Risk of bias (Design/ Risk of bias)	Consistency	Directness	Precision	Magnitude of effect	High, Moderate, Low, Insufficient
Intensive Care Plus Outreach versus Standard Care (Hawton 2000 as cited in Mann 2005)[10]						
Unclear outcome reported in Mann 2005						
1 systematic review; not reported	Medium (SR/Unclear)	N/A	Indirect	N/A	Not reported	Insufficient to Low

Table 8. Intensive Case Management

| Number of studies; # of subjects | Domains pertaining to strength of evidence | | | | Magnitude of effect | Strength of evidence |
	Risk of bias (Design/ Risk of bias)	Consistency	Directness	Precision	Summary effect size (95% CI)	High, Moderate, Low, Insufficient
Intensive Case Management versus Treatment as Usual (De Leo 2007)[45]						
Suicide at 12 months						
1; 22	High (RCT/High)	N/A	Indirect	Imprecise	No suicides in either group	Insufficient
Self-harming behavior at 6 months						
1; 22	High (RCT/High)	N/A	Indirect	Imprecise	Intensive case management: 3/14 (21.4%) Treatment as usual: 1/8 (12.4%) 12 months:	Insufficient
Self-harming behavior at 12 months						
1; 22	High (RCT/High)	N/A	Indirect	Imprecise	Intensive case management: 2/14 (14.3%) Treatment as usual: 2/8 (25.0%)	Insufficient

Table 9. Interpersonal Psychotherapy

| Number of studies; # of subjects | Domains pertaining to strength of evidence | | | | Magnitude of effect | Strength of evidence |
	Risk of bias (Design/ Risk of bias)	Consistency	Directness	Precision	Magnitude of effect	High, Moderate, Low, Insufficient
Interpersonal Psychotherapy versus Standard Care (Guthrie 2001 as cited in Mann 2005)[10]						
Unclear outcome reported in Mann 2005						
1; not reported	Medium (RCT/Unclear)	N/A	Indirect	N/A	Not reported	Insufficient to Low

Table 10. Mentalization Based Treatment (MBT)

| Number of studies; # of subjects | Domains pertaining to strength of evidence | | | | Magnitude of effect | Strength of evidence |
	Risk of bias (Design/ Risk of bias)	Consistency	Directness	Precision	Magnitude of effect	High, Moderate, Low, Insufficient
MBT versus treatment as usual (Bateman 2008)						
Any suicide attempt						
1; 41	High (RCT/High)	N/A	Indirect	Imprecise	d=2.0 (95% CI, 1.4 to 4.9)	Insufficient
Mean total suicide attempts						
1; 41	High (RCT/High)	N/A	Indirect	Imprecise	d=1.4 (95% CI, 1.3 to 1.5)	Insufficient
MBT versus Structured Clinical Management (SCM) (Bateman 2009)[37]						
Life-threatening suicide attempts, proportion with episode at end of treatment						
1; 134	Medium (RCT/Unclear)	N/A	Indirect	Imprecise	d=0.65 (95% CI, 0.58 to 0.73)	Low
Severe self-harm incidents, proportion with episode at end of treatment						
1; 134	Medium (RCT/Unclear)	N/A	Indirect	Imprecise	d=0.62 (95% CI, 0.28 to 0.97)	Low

Table 11. Personal Construct Psychotherapy

Number of studies; # of subjects	Domains pertaining to strength of evidence				Magnitude of effect	Strength of evidence
	Risk of bias (Design/ Risk of bias)	Consistency	Directness	Precision	Magnitude of effect	High, Moderate, Low, Insufficient
Personal Construct Psychotherapy versus Normal Clinical Practice (Winter 2007)[43]						
Deaths by suicide after 5 years						
1; 40	High (RCT/High)	N/A	Indirect	Imprecise	PCP = 1; NCP = 2; p not reported	Insufficient
Repetition of deliberate self-harm after 5 years						
1; 40	High (RCT/High)	N/A	Indirect	Imprecise	39% vs 58% (P=0.15)	Insufficient

Table 12. Problem-Solving Therapy

Number of studies; # of subjects	Domains pertaining to strength of evidence				Magnitude of effect	Strength of evidence
	Risk of bias (Design/ Risk of bias)	Consistency	Directness	Precision	Magnitude of effect	High, Moderate, Low, Insufficient
Problem-Solving Therapy plus treatment as usual versus treatment as usual (Hatcher 2011)[36]						
Participants re-presenting to hospital for self-harm: All consenting patients						
1; 552	Low (RCT/Low)	N/A	Indirect	Imprecise	RR= 0.17 (95% CI -0.24 to 0.44); P=0.43	Moderate
Participants with self-reported self-harm: All consenting patients						
1; 412	Low (RCT/Low)	N/A	Indirect	Imprecise	RR= 0.16 (95% CI -0.13 to 0.38); P=0.29	Moderate
Time to re-presentation to hospital for self-harm: All consenting patients						
1; 139	Low (RCT/Low)	N/A	Indirect	Imprecise	HR= 0.81 (95% CI 0.53 to 1.25); P=0.92	Moderate
Participants re-presenting to hospital for self-harm: Consenting patients; first episode of self-harm hospitalization is index episode						
1; 306	Low (RCT/Low)	N/A	Indirect	Imprecise	RR= -0.56 (95% CI -1.96 to 0.18); P=0.23	Moderate
Participants with self-reported self-harm: Consenting patients; first episode of self-harm hospitalization is index episode						
1; 220	Low (RCT/Low)	N/A	Indirect	Imprecise	RR= -0.25 (95% CI -1.03 to 0.24); P=0.47	Moderate
Time to re-presentation to hospital for self-harm: Consenting patients; first episode of self-harm hospitalization is index episode						
1; 137	Low (RCT/Low)	N/A	Indirect	Imprecise	HR= 1.62 (95% CI 0.82 to 3.18); P=0.16	Moderate
Participants re-presenting to hospital for self-harm: Consenting patients; repeat episode of self-harm hospitalization is index episode						
1; 246	Low (RCT/Low)	N/A	Indirect	Imprecise	RR= 0.47 (95% CI 0.11 to 0.69); P=0.02; NNT=8	Moderate
Participants with self-reported self-harm: Consenting patients; repeat episode of self-harm hospitalization is index episode						
1; 192	Low (RCT/Low)	N/A	Indirect	Imprecise	RR= 0.37 (95% CI 0.08 to 0.57); P=0.02; NNT=6	Moderate

Time to re-presentation to hospital for self-harm: Consenting patients; repeat episode of self-harm hospitalization is index episode						
1; 149	Low (RCT/Low)	N/A	Indirect	Imprecise	HR= 0.47 (95% CI 0.26 to 0.85); P=0.01	Moderate
Participants re-presenting to hospital for self-harm: All patients						
1; 1094	Low (RCT/Low)	N/A	Indirect	Imprecise	RR= 0.05 (95% CI -0.28 to 0.30); P=0.79	Moderate
Time to re-presentation to hospital for self-harm: All patients						
1; 149	Low (RCT/Low)	N/A	Indirect	Imprecise	HR= 0.98 (95% CI 0.71 to 1.36); P=0.92	Moderate
Participants re-presenting to hospital for self-harm: All patients; first episode of self-harm hospitalization is index episode						
1; 674	Low (RCT/Low)	N/A	Indirect	Imprecise	RR= 0.42 (95% CI -1.17 to 0.08); P=0.37	Moderate
Time to re-presentation to hospital for self-harm: All patients; first episode of self-harm hospitalization is index episode						
1; 135	Low (RCT/Low)	N/A	Indirect	Imprecise	HR= 1.55 (95% CI 0.98 to 2.48); P=0.06	Moderate
Participants re-presenting to hospital for self-harm: All patients; repeat episode of self-harm hospitalization is index episode						
1; 420	Low (RCT/Low)	N/A	Indirect	Imprecise	RR= 0.39 (95% CI 0.07 to 0.60); P=0.03; NNT=12	Moderate
Time to re-presentation to hospital for self-harm: All patients; repeat episode of self-harm hospitalization is index episode						
1; 194	Low (RCT/Low)	N/A	Indirect	Imprecise	HR= 0.58 (95% CI 0.36 to 0.94); P=0.03	Moderate
Problem-Solving Therapy versus Standard Care (Hawton 2000 as cited in Mann 2005)[10]						
Unclear outcome reported in Mann 2005						
1 systematic review; not reported	Medium (SR/Unclear)	N/A	Indirect	N/A	Not reported	Insufficient to Low
CBT vs Problem Solving Therapy vs Usual Care (Stewart 2009)[50] Repeated in Cognitive Therapy table above						
Average number of suicide attempts						
1; 32	High (RCT/High)	N/A	Indirect	Imprecise	CBT: 0.22 PST: 0.33 TAU: 0.22 No significant differences found for repetition of suicide attempts when PST group was compared to TAU	Insufficient

Table 13. Psychoanalytically Oriented Partial Hospitalization

	Domains pertaining to strength of evidence				Magnitude of effect	Strength of evidence
Number of studies; # of subjects	**Risk of bias (Design/ Risk of bias)**	**Consistency**	**Directness**	**Precision**	**Magnitude of effect**	**High, Moderate, Low, Insufficient**
Psychoanalytically Oriented Partial Hospitalization versus Standard Care in patients with Borderline Personality Disorder (Bateman 2001 as cited in Mann 2005)[10]						
Unclear outcome reported in Mann 2005						
1; not reported	Medium (RCT/Unclear)	N/A	Indirect	N/A	Not reported	Insufficient to Low

Table 14. Skills Based Treatment

Number of studies; # of subjects	Domains pertaining to strength of evidence				Magnitude of effect	Strength of evidence
	Risk of bias (Design/ Risk of bias)	Consistency	Directness	Precision	Magnitude of effect	High, Moderate, Low, Insufficient
Skills Based Treatment versus Supportive Relationship Treatment (Donaldson 2005)[48]						
Number of re-attempts at 6 months						
1; 39	High (RCT/High)	N/A	Indirect	Imprecise	SBT=26.7% (4/15) vs SRT=12.5% (2/16); χ2=1.00	Insufficient

Table 15. Systems Training for Emotional Predictability and Problem Solving (STEPPS)

Number of studies; # of subjects	Domains pertaining to strength of evidence				Magnitude of effect	Strength of evidence
	Risk of bias (Design/ Risk of bias)	Consistency	Directness	Precision	Magnitude of effect	High, Moderate, Low, Insufficient
Systems Training for Emotional Predictability and Problem Solving versus treatment as usual (Blum 2008)[39]						
Time to first suicide attempt						
1; 165	High (RCT/High)	N/A	Indirect	Imprecise	χ2<0.1, df=1, p=0.994	Low
Time to first self-harm act						
1; 165	High (RCT/High)	N/A	Indirect	Imprecise	χ2<0.1, df=1, p=0.902	Low

[a] This review did not evaluate any outcomes other than suicidal self-directed violence, and therefore no additional data on potential harms and side effects was investigated. Potential harms and side effects should always be considered when evaluating the strength of evidence and considering adoption of an intervention or referral/follow-up service.

APPENDIX T. QUALITY RATING OF SYSTEMATIC REVIEWS RELATED TO REFERRAL/ FOLLOW-UP SERVICES USING OXMAN AND GUYATT[15] CRITERIA

Author Year of systematic review	Search methods reported	Comprehensive search	Inclusion criteria reported	Selection bias avoided	Validity criteria reported	Validity assessed appropriately	Methods used to combine studies reported	Findings combined appropriately	Conclusions supported by data	Overall scientific quality (higher score is better)
Dieterich 2010[106]	Yes	Yes; only searched one database, though this database combines multiple other databases	Yes	Yes	Yes	Yes	Yes	Yes	Yes	7
Hailey 2008[118]	Yes	Yes	Yes	Yes	Yes	Yes	Yes	Can't tell	Yes	6
Innamorati 2011[90]	Yes	No; no hand-searching, reference list searching, or asking experts noted	Partially; very general statement re: inclusion	No	Yes	Partially/Can't tell; sometimes did, but often didn't	No	Yes	Yes	3
Lapierre 2011[109]	Yes	Yes	Yes	Can't tell; detailed results of study selection not reported, no reasons for exclusions described	Yes	No; reported validity assessment, but did not do any type of analysis with it	Yes	Yes	Yes	5
Newton 2010[112]	Yes	Yes	Yes	Yes	Yes	Yes	Yes	Yes	Yes	7
Shekelle 2009[14] & Bagley 2010[103]	Yes	Yes	Yes	Yes	Yes	Yes	Yes	Yes	Yes	7
Soomro 2008[96]	Yes	No; no hand-searching, reference list searching, or asking experts noted	Yes	No	Yes	Yes	No	Yes	Yes	4

Author Year of systematic review	Search methods reported	Comprehensive search	Inclusion criteria reported	Selection bias avoided	Validity criteria reported	Validity assessed appropriately	Methods used to combine studies reported	Findings combined appropriately	Conclusions supported by data	Overall scientific quality (higher score is better)
State of Victoria Department of Health 2010[115]	Yes	No; no hand-searching, reference list searching, or asking experts noted	Yes	Yes	Yes	Yes	Yes	Can't tell	Yes	6
van der Feltz-Cornelis 2011[119]	Yes	Yes	Yes	Yes	Yes	Yes	Yes	Yes	Can't tell. For example, awareness campaigns are categorized as actually or potentially effective in the Discussion. But, in Table 2, the Effect Sizes include "no detectable effect", "no effect", and "inconclusive"	5

APPENDIX U. DATA ABSTRACTION OF PRIMARY STUDIES OBTAINED FROM GOOD QUALITY SYSTEMATIC REVIEWS RELATED TO REFERRAL/FOLLOW-UP SERVICES

Author Year of systematic review	Time period and databases searched in systematic review	Eligibility criteria in systematic review	Study designs of eligible studies	Countries included in eligible studies	Sample size in eligible studies	Population in eligible studies	Interventions in eligible studies	Main results of eligible studies
Dieterich 2010[106]	Cochrane Schizophrenia Group Trials Registry: database inception through February 2009	Randomized clinical trial, focused on people with severe mental illness, ages 18-65 years, community care setting, intensive case management (ICM) compared to non-intensive case management or standard care	One RCT: Killaspy 2006[58]	UK	251	People with severe mental illness, mean age was 39 years (SD 11); 58% male; 36% Afro-Caribbean	ICM Assertive Community Treatment versus non-ICM Community Mental Health Treatment	One out of 127 patients assigned to ICM and three out of 124 patients assigned to non-ICM died by suicide; 10 ICM and 13 non-ICM patients ($p = 0.40$) engaged in deliberate self-harm including suicide.
Hailey 2008[118]	MEDLINE, HealthSTAR, EMBASE, PsycINFO, CINAHL, ACP Journal Club, CDSR, DARE, CCRCT: to June 2006	Clinical or administrative outcomes of Telemental Health applications; controlled studies comparing Telemental Health to a non-Telemental Health alternative; non-controlled studies with no fewer than 20 subjects	No eligible RCTs	No eligible RCTs	No eligible RCTs	No eligible RCTs	No eligible RCTs	No eligible RCTs
Newton 2010[112]	MEDLINE, EMBASE, CCRCT, HealthStar, CDSR, Health Technology Assessment Database, DARE, Academic Search Elite, PsycINFO, Health Source: Nursing and Academic Edition, CINAHL, SocIndex, ProQuest Theses and Dissertations, Child Welfare Information Gateway: 1985-October 2009	Experimental or quasi-experimental designs; mental health-based, suicide-prevention-focused intervention initiated in the ED or immediately after ED discharge through direct referral/enrollment; children and adolescents (aged ≤18 years), or their parents or ED personnel; at least one clinically relevant primary outcome	No eligible RCTs	No eligible RCTs	No eligible RCTs	No eligible RCTs	No eligible RCTs	No eligible RCTs

Author Year of systematic review	Time period and databases searched in systematic review	Eligibility criteria in systematic review	Study designs of eligible studies	Countries included in eligible studies	Sample size in eligible studies	Population in eligible studies	Interventions in eligible studies	Main results of eligible studies
Shekelle 2009[14] & Bagley 2010[103]	MEDLINE, Cochrane Library, PsycINFO: June 2005-May 2008	English language, suicide or suicide attempt outcomes, no mental health interventions such as psychotherapy or pharmacotherapy interventions unless they included Veterans	One RCT: Carter 2005[54]	Australia	772	Non-Veteran/ Military; no other data reported	Postcards mailed every 1-2 months for a year post-discharge	57 repeated self-harm incidents in the treatment group compared to 68 incidents in the control group
State of Victoria Department of Health 2010[115]	MEDLINE, EMBASE, AMED, PsycINFO: January 1997-February 2009	English language, human, suicide related outcome, sample size ≥6, no duplication, emergency department or other acute care setting	One RCT reported in 2 papers: Carter 2005[54] Carter 2007[55]	Australia	772	Mean age 33 years for treatment group, 34 years for control; patients had an average of 2 psychiatric diagnoses	Postcards mailed every 1-2 months for a year post-discharge	RR 0.55, 95% CI 0.35-0.87 for repeat episodes of self-poisoning at 12 months follow-up; RR 0.49, 95% CI 0.33-0.73 for repeat episodes of self-poisoning at 24 months

APPENDIX V. SUMMARY OF SYSTEMATIC REVIEW RESULTS RELATED TO REFERRAL AND FOLLOW-UP SERVICES FROM GAYNES ET AL., MANN ET AL., AND NICE REVIEWS[9-11]

	Gaynes 2004[9]	Mann 2005[10]	NICE 2011[11]
Overall conclusions	The poor generalizability of the studies makes the overall strength of evidence fair, at best, while the results are mixed. Although some trends suggest incremental benefit from several interventions, no consistent statistically significant effects have emerged for interventions for which more than one study has been done.	Interventions need more evidence of efficacy.	Compared with usual care, there was insufficient evidence to determine clinical effects between interventions and routine care in the reduction of the proportion of patients who repeated self-harm. Thus, no conclusions could be made regarding psychosocial interventions on reduction of repetitions of self-harm. For the outcome of suicide, no conclusions could be drawn due to the small evidence base.
Scope			
Search dates	1966-October 2002	1966-June 2005	Up to January 2011
Populations included	Population of interest was primary care patients with previously unidentified suicide risk. Included RCTs were conducted in high-risk groups as identified by a deliberate self-harm episode, diagnosis of borderline personality disorder, or admission to a psychiatric unit.	Not specified	Adults, children, and young people with previous self-harm behavior
Interventions included	Pharmacotherapy, psychotherapy, referral/follow-up	Pharmacotherapy, psychotherapy, referral/follow-up	Pharmacotherapy, psychotherapy, referral/follow-up
Suicide-related outcomes included	Suicide completions, suicide attempts	Completed and attempted suicide	Primary outcome was repetition of self-harm; also included suicide outcomes.
Settings/countries included	Primary or specialty care settings; no exclusions based on country.	Included settings not specified; no exclusions based on country.	No exclusions by country
Other exclusion criteria	Clinical trials targeting patients with chronic psychotic illnesses; studies without adequate comparison groups.	No additional exclusion criteria specified.	
Main Results: Referral and Follow-up Services			
Emergency contact card	Fewer suicide attempts		Insufficient evidence for repeat self-harm and suicide prevention.
Intensive care plus outreach	Meta-analysis of 6 studies produced a non-significant result in terms of decreasing repetition of deliberate self-harm.		
Intensive psychosocial follow-up		No benefit in terms of re-attempt rate when compared to standard care.	
Postal contact	No benefit	Fewer suicides	Insufficient evidence for repeat self-harm; possible suicide prevention effect should be interpreted with caution.
Telephone follow-up	No benefit	No benefit in terms of re-attempt rate when compared to standard care.	Insufficient evidence for repeat self-harm and suicide prevention.
24-hour access to contact with a mental health professional	Trend toward decreasing repetition of self-harm in one RCT		

APPENDIX W. DESCRIPTION OF PRIMARY OUTCOMES AND INTENT TO TREAT SUICIDAL SELF-DIRECTED VIOLENCE FOR STUDIES RELATED TO REFERRAL AND FOLLOW-UP SERVICES

Study, Year	Designed to treat suicide? (yes/no/unclear)	N	Outcome definition	Results
Beautrais 2010[53]	Yes; study aim was to test effectiveness of intervention to reduce self-harm re-presentations	327	Re-presentations for self-harm were assessed by monitoring psychiatric emergency service records and hospital medical records were reviewed at the conclusion of the 12-month follow-up period. Three measures of re-presentation were calculated from these data: re-presentations to psychiatric emergency service, re-presentations to Christchurch Hospital emergency department and total re-presentations to either the psychiatric emergency service or emergency department	Unadjusted analyses: Re-presentation for self-harm, %: To psychiatric emergency service: PC=15.0 vs TAU=23.6, P<0.06, OR= 0.57 (95% CI, 0.33 to 1.01) To emergency department: PC=25.5 vs TAU=27.0, P>0.75; OR=0.92 (95% CI 0.56 to 1.52) Total (psychiatric emergency service or emergency department): PC=25.5vs TAU=28.2, P>0.58, OR=0.87 (95% CI 0.53 to 1.43) Number of self-harm re-presentations: To psychiatric emergency service: PC=23.5 vs TAU=51.1, P<0.0001, IRR= 0.46 (95% CI, 0.31 to 0.68) To emergency department: PC=53.6 vs TAU=71.8, P<0.04, IRR= 0.75 (95% CI, 0.56 to 0.99) Total (psychiatric emergency service or emergency department): PC=56.9 vs TAU=78.2, P<0.03; IRR=0.73 (95% CI, 0.56 to 0.95) Analyses adjusted for prior self-harm Re-presentation for self-harm, % To psychiatric emergency service: PC=16.2 vs TAU= 22.5; P>0.13; OR=0.64 (95% CI, 0.36 to 1.15) To emergency department: PC=26.6 vs TAU= 26.0; P>0.88; OR=1.04 (95% CI, 0.62 to 1.73) Total (psychiatric emergency service or emergency department): PC=26.6 vs TAU=27.2; P>0.91; OR=0.97 (95% CI, 0.58 to 1.62) Number of self-harm re-presentations To psychiatric emergency service: PC=28.7 vs TAU=44.1; P>0.04; IRR=0.65 (95% CI, 0.43 to 0.98) To emergency department: PC=67.2 vs TAU=61.0; P>0.52; IRR=1.10 (95% CI, 0.82 to 1.49) Total (psychiatric emergency service or emergency department): PC=71.1 vs TAU=66.4; P>0.64; IRR=1.07 (95% CI, 0.80 to 1.43)
Carter 2005[54]	Yes; primary outcome was repeat self poisoning.	772	Proportion of patients with at least one repeat episode of deliberate self poisoning in 24 months and the number of repeat episodes of deliberate self poisoning per individual over 24 months	12-month outcomes Proportion of patients with repeat deliberate self poisoning: PC=57 (15.1%, 95% CI 11.5% to 18.7%) vs TAU=68 (17.3%, 95% CI, 13.5% to 21%); difference between groups -2% (95% CI, -7% to 3%); χ2=0.675, df = 1, P = 0.41 Cumulative number of repeat episodes of deliberate self poisoning: PC=101 vs TAU=192 Risk of repetition= overall incidence risk ratio (IRR) 0.55 (95% CI, 0.35 to 0.87); men only: IRR= 0.97 (95% CI, 0.48 to 1.98); women only: IRR= 0.54 (95% CI, 0.30 to 0.96) 24-month outcomes Proportion of patients with repeat deliberate self poisoning: PC=21.2% (80/378; 95% CI, 17.0 to 25.3) vs TAU=22.8% (90/394; 95% CI, 18.7 to 27.0); difference between groups -1.7% (95% CI, -7.5 to 4.2); χ2=0.317, df = 1, P = 0.57 Cumulative number of repeat episodes of deliberate self poisoning: PC=145 vs TAU=310 Risk of repetition= overall IRR 0.49 (95% CI, 0.33 to 0.73); men only: IRR= 0.97 (95% CI, 0.50 to 1.88); women only: IRR= 0.49 (95% CI, 0.30 to 0.80)

Study, Year	Designed to treat suicide? (yes/no/unclear)	N	Outcome definition	Results
Gallo 2007 (PROSPECT)[59]	Unclear; states that PROSPECT was an effectiveness study designed to assess the effect of care management on reducing risk factors for late-life suicide, but the primary outcome in this study was mortality, not suicide specifically	599	National Center for Health Statistics National Death Index (NDI) Plus was used to assess vital status over a 5-year period. The underlying causes of death obtained from NDI Plus are similar to codes assigned by trained nosologists (Doody 2001, Sathiakumar 1998)	Suicide N, n/1000 person-years (95% CI) All patients (N=599): IG=1, 0.7 (0.0 to 4.2) vs UC=0, 0.0 (0.0 to 3.3) Patients with major depression disorder (N=396): IG=0, 0.0 (0.0 to 4.1) vs UC=0, 0.0 (0.0 to 5.1) Patients with clinically significant minor depression (n =203): IG=1, 2.2 (0.1 to 2.5) vs UC=0, 0.0 (0.0 to 9.7) Patients without depression (n=627): IG=0, 0.0 (0.0 to 3.0) vs UC=0, 0.0 (0.0 to 2.5)
Killaspy 2006 (REACT)[58]	Yes; secondary outcomes included serious incidents concerning deliberate self-harm	251	Serious incidents concerning deliberate self-harm during the 18-month study period. Outcome criteria were not reported.	Committed suicide: ACT=0.8% (1/124) vs CMH=2.5% (3/119); between-groups comparison not reported Deliberate self-harm: ACT=8% (10/91) vs CMH=11% (13/75); mean difference= 0.72; P=0.40
King 2006[57]	Yes; outcome measures included the Spectrum of Suicide Behavior Scale (Pfeffer, 1986); a 5-point rating of history of suicidality (none, ideation, intent/threat, mild attempt, serious attempt).	236	Suicide attempts were measured through self-report on the Spectrum of Suicide Behavior Scale (Pfeffer, 1986)	No significant differences between groups in percent of adolescents with one or more suicide attempts % with 1 or more suicide attempts during the 6 month follow-up: TAU=11.7, TAU+YST-1=18.1% (fishers exact test, P=.22)
King 2009[56]	Yes; the presence or absence of one or more suicide attempts during each follow-up period was assessed with an item from the NIMH DISC-IV Mood Disorders module.	346	Presence or absence of one or more suicide attempts during follow-up was assessed via self-report, using the question, "Have you tried to kill yourself?" from the NIMH DISC-IV Mood Disorders Module.	No significant differences were found between groups for percent of adolescents with one or more attempts. % with one or more attempts in the 12 month follow-up period: TAU=35, TAU+YST-II=29, Chi-square (1, N=354)=0.66, p=.42 One suicide death occurred in the TAU group, no suicide deaths in the TAU+YST-II group

APPENDIX X. DATA ABSTRACTION FOR PRIMARY STUDIES RELATED TO REFERRAL/FOLLOW-UP SERVICES

Author, Year (Country):	Beautrais 2010[53] (New Zealand)
Population:	All individuals aged 16 and older who presented to psychiatric emergency services at Christchurch Hospital, New Zealand, following self-harm or attempted suicide during the period 1 August 2006 to 6 April 2007.
Intervention 1:	Treatment as usual (TAU) consisted of crisis assessment and referral to in-patient community-based mental health services.
Intervention 2:	TAU plus postcard intervention (PC), which consisted of a series of six 'postcards' sent by mail during the 12 months following the participant's index presentation for suicide attempt or self-harm. The postcard read: 'It has been a short time since you were here at PES (Psych Emergency), and we hope things are going well for you. If you wish to drop us a note we would be happy to hear from you'. Postcards were printed on A4 paper and posted in a plain sealed envelope to the participant's residential address. Postcards were posted at the following times after the index presentation: 2 and 6 weeks; 3, 6, 9 and 12 months.
Setting:	Acute psychiatric emergency services, serving a population of approximately 500,000 people
N:	327; PC=153, TAU=174
Mean age, % female, race (variance):	Age, years (variance NR): PC=33.8 vs TAU=33.9 % female: PC=70.4% vs TAU=62.3% Race NR
Outcome assessment:	Re-presentations for self-harm were assessed by monitoring psychiatric emergency service records and hospital medical records were reviewed at the conclusion of the 12-month follow-up period. Three measures of re-presentation were calculated from these data: re-presentations to psychiatric emergency service, re-presentations to Christchurch Hospital emergency department and total re-presentations to either the psychiatric emergency service or emergency department.
Results:	Unadjusted analyses: *Re-presentation for self-harm, %:* To psychiatric emergency service: PC=15.0 vs TAU=23.6, $P<0.06$, OR= 0.57 (95% CI, 0.33 to 1.01) To emergency department: PC=25.5 vs TAU=27.0, $P>0.75$; OR=0.92 (95% CI 0.56 to 1.52) Total (psychiatric emergency service or emergency department): PC=25.5vs TAU=28.2, $P>0.58$, OR=0.87 (95% CI 0.53 to 1.43) *Number of self-harm re-presentations:* To psychiatric emergency service: PC=23.5 vs TAU=51.1, $P<0.0001$, IRR= 0.46 (95% CI, 0.31 to 0.68) To emergency department: PC=53.6 vs TAU=71.8, $P<0.04$, IRR= 0.75 (95% CI, 0.56 to 0.99) Total (psychiatric emergency service or emergency department): PC=56.9 vs TAU=78.2, $P<0.03$; IRR=0.73 (95% CI, 0.56 to 0.95) Analyses adjusted for prior self-harm *Re-presentation for self-harm, %* To psychiatric emergency service: PC=16.2 vs TAU= 22.5; $P>0.13$; OR=0.64 (95% CI, 0.36 to 1.15) To emergency department: PC=26.6 vs TAU= 26.0; $P>0.88$; OR=1.04 (95% CI, 0.62 to 1.73) Total (psychiatric emergency service or emergency department): PC=26.6 vs TAU=27.2; $P>0.91$; OR=0.97 (95% CI, 0.58 to 1.62) *Number of self-harm re-presentations* To psychiatric emergency service: PC=28.7 vs TAU=44.1; $P>0.04$; IRR=0.65 (95% CI, 0.43 to 0.98) To emergency department: PC=67.2 vs TAU=61.0; $P>0.52$; IRR=1.10 (95% CI, 0.82 to 1.49) Total (psychiatric emergency service or emergency department): PC=71.1 vs TAU=66.4; $P>0.64$; IRR=1.07 (95% CI, 0.80 to 1.43)

Author, Year (Country):	Carter 2005[54] – 12-month outcomes Carter 2007[55] – 24-month outcomes (Australia)
Population:	Those aged over 16 years who presented with deliberate self poisoning during April 1998 to December 2001 to the Hunter Area Toxicology Service at the Newcastle Mater Hospital, New South Wales, Australia, which serves a primary referral population of 385 000 adults and a tertiary referral population of a further 170 000
Intervention 1:	Treatment as usual (TAU); no details provided
Intervention 2:	A postcard (PC) sent to participants in a sealed envelope at 1, 2, 3, 4, 6, 8, 10, and 12 months after discharge, plus TAU
Setting:	Not specified
N:	772: PC=378 vs TAU=394
Mean age, % female, race (variance):	Median age, years (interquartile range): 33 (24-44) 68% female Race not reported
Other clinical characteristics:	17% previous admission for deliberate self-poisoning Median number of psychiatric diagnoses (interquartile range): 2 (1-2)
Outcome assessment:	Proportion of patients with at least one repeat episode of deliberate self poisoning in 24 months and the number of repeat episodes of deliberate self poisoning per individual over 24 months
Results:	12-month outcomes: Proportion of patients with repeat deliberate self poisoning: PC=57 (15.1%, 95% CI 11.5% to 18.7%) vs TAU=68 (17.3%, 95% CI, 13.5% to 21%); difference between groups -2% (95% CI, -7% to 3%); χ^2=0.675, df = 1, $P = 0.41$ Cumulative number of repeat episodes of deliberate self poisoning: PC=101 vs TAU=192 Risk of repetition= overall incidence risk ratio (IRR) 0.55 (95% CI, 0.35 to 0.87); men only: IRR= 0.97 (95% CI, 0.48 to 1.98; women only: IRR= 0.54 (95% CI, 0.30 to 0.96) 24-month outcomes Proportion of patients with repeat deliberate self poisoning: PC=21.2% (80/378; 95% CI, 17.0 to 25.3) vs TAU=22.8% (90/394; 95% CI, 18.7 to 27.0); difference between groups -1.7% (95% CI, -7.5 to 4.2); χ^2=0. 317, df = 1, $P = 0.57$ Cumulative number of repeat episodes of deliberate self poisoning: PC=145 vs TAU=310 Risk of repetition= overall IRR 0.49 (95% CI, 0.33 to 0.73); men only: IRR= 0.49 (95% CI, 0.30 to 0.80); women only: IRR= 0.49 (95% CI, 0.50 to 1.88)

Author, Year (Country):	PROSPECT (Prevention of Suicide in Primary Care Elderly: Collaborative Trial) (US) Gallo 2007[59]: 5-year outcomes Bruce 2004[120], Schulberg 2001[127]: Additional detail on methods
Population:	Age ≥ 60 years and score greater than 20 on the Centers for Epidemiologic Studies Depression scale
Therapy 1:	Usual Care (UC): Practices received educational sessions for primary care physicians and notification of the depression status of their patients, but no specific recommendations were given to physicians about individual patients, except for psychiatric emergencies.
Therapy 2:	Intervention Group (IG): On-site depression care manager working with primary care physicians to provide algorithm-based care. Depression care manager's role included (1) obtaining needed clinical information from the patient and prompting the physician with timely and targeted recommendations about appropriate care of the patient's depression; (2) monitoring patient's clinical course and encouraging adherence; (3) educating patients, families and physicians on depression and suicidal ideation.

Author, Year (Country):	PROSPECT (Prevention of Suicide in Primary Care Elderly: Collaborative Trial) (US) Gallo 2007[59]: 5-year outcomes Bruce 2004[120], Schulberg 2001[127]: Additional detail on methods
Medication regimen:	All patients received citalopram, initiated at 10 mg before bedtime on the first day, 20 mg/d for the next 6 days, and 30 mg/d subsequently. After 6 weeks, the target dosage was maintained if the patient exhibited a substantial improvement ($\geq$ 50% reduction in the HDRS or was increased if the patient exhibited a partial improvement (30% to 50% reduction in the HDRS score). Nonresponders, for whom guidelines called for switching to another antidepressant, were defined as patients who did not demonstrate either minimal improvement after 6 weeks of treatment at the target dosage or substantial improvement after the dose was increased to the maximum recommended dose after 12 weeks of treatment For patients who had not responded at 12 weeks, the health specialist followed guidelines for switching antidepressants.
Setting:	20 primary care practices; 16 community-based and 4 were academic practices
Therapist characteristics:	The 15 care managers included social workers, nurses, and psychologists
Treatment duration:	12 months
N:	599; IG=320, UC=279
Mean age, % female, race (variance):	Mean age (SD): IG=71 (7.8) vs UC=70 (8.1) % female: IG=69% vs UC=75% Ethnic minority (Hispanic, non-Hispanic Black, Asian, other non-Hispanic): IG=29% vs UC=37%
Other clinical characteristics:	Mean MMSE score for cognitive function (SD): IG= 27 (2.9) vs UC= 27 (2.5) Major depressive disorder: IG=67% vs UC=65% Mean Hamilton Depression Rating Scale score for depression severity (SD): IG=19 (6.1) vs UC=18 (5.8) % with Scale for Suicidal Ideation score >0): IG= 29% vs UC=20%
Concomitant medications:	4 months: Medication and psychotherapy: IG=5.8% vs UC=8.5%; OR 0.46 (95% CI, 0.13 to1.66) Medication only: IG=57.7% vs UC=40.4%; OR 4.91 (95% CI, 2.13 to 11.33) 8 months: Medication and psychotherapy: IG=9.7% vs UC=8.9%; OR 1.29 (95% CI, 0.39 to 4.30) Medication only: IG=57.0% vs UC=39.4%; OR 4.20 (95% CI, 1.77 to 9.96) 12 months: Medication and psychotherapy: IG=6.8% vs UC=13.6%; OR 0.25 (95% CI, 0.07 to 0.96) Medication only: IG=66.3% vs UC=44.2%; OR 7.21 (95% CI, 2.86 to 18.18)
Outcome assessment:	National Center for Health Statistics NDI Plus was used to assess vital status over a 5-year period. The underlying causes of death that we obtained from NDI Plus are similar to codes assigned by trained nosologists (Doody 2001, Sathiakumar 1998)
Results:	Suicide N, n/1000 person-years (95% CI) All patients (N=599): IG=1, 0.7 (0.0 to 4.2) vs UC=0, 0.0 (0.0 to 3.3) Patients with major depression disorder (N=396): IG=0, 0.0 (0.0 to 4.1) vs UC=0, 0.0 (0.0 to 5.1) Patients with clinically significant minor depression (n =203): IG=1, 2.2 (0.1 to 2.5) vs UC=0, 0.0 (0.0 to 9.7) Patients without depression (n=627): IG=0, 0.0 (0.0 to 3.0) vs UC=0, 0.0 (0.0 to 2.5)

Author, Year (Country):	REACT study (Randomized Evaluation of Assertive Community Treatment) (UK) Killaspy 2006[58]
Population:	People living in independent or low supported accommodations; under the care of the community mental health team for at least 12 months and identified as having difficulty engaging with standard community care; primary diagnosis of serious mental illness (for example, schizophrenia, schizoaffective disorder, other chronic psychosis, bipolar affective disorder); and recent high use of inpatient care (at least 100 consecutive inpatient days or at least five admissions within the past two years or at least 50 consecutive inpatient days or at least three admissions within the past year)
Therapy 1:	Assertive community treatment (ACT): Total team case load=80 to 100; maximum individual case load=12; availability=extended hours (0800 to 2000 every day); locations for appointments=not office based ("in vivo"): meet client at home, in cafes, parks, etc; contact with clients=assertive engagement: multiple attempts, flexible and various approaches (for example, befriending, offering practical support, leisure activities); commitment to care="no drop-out" policy: continue to try to engage in long term care; case work style=team approach—all team members work with all clients; Frequency of team meetings=frequent (up to daily) to discuss clients and daily plans; source of skills=team rather than outside agencies as far as possible
Therapy 2:	Community mental health (CMH): Total team case load=300 to 350; maximum individual case load=35; availability=office hours only (0900 to 1700 Mon–Fri); locations for appointments=office based appointments and home visits; contact with clients=offer appointments at office or make home visits; commitment to care=discharge if unable to make or maintain contact; case work style=case management—little "sharing" of work with clients between team members; frequency of team meetings=weekly; source of skills="brokerage": referral to outside agencies for advice (for example, social security benefits, housing)
Medication regimen:	Not reported
Setting:	See 'location for appointment' information for each therapy, respectively
Therapist characteristics:	Not reported
Treatment duration:	18 months
N:	251: ACT=127 vs CMH=124
Mean age, % female, race (variance):	Mean age, years (SD): ACT=38 (11) vs CMH=40 (11) % female: ACT=38% vs CMH=45% % White: ACT=51% vs CMH=57% % African Caribbean: ACT=41% vs CMH=31% % Other Race: ACT=8% vs CMH=11%
Other clinical characteristics:	% patients: Schizophrenia: ACT=68% vs CMH=65% Schizoaffective: ACT=17% vs CMH=15% Bipolar affective: ACT=6% vs CMH=4% Delusional disorder: ACT=3% vs CMH=5% Major depression: ACT=0 vs CMH=2% Other diagnoses: ACT=6% vs CMH=8%
Concomitant medications:	Not reported
Outcome assessment:	Serious incidents concerning deliberate self-harm during the 18-month study period. Outcome criteria were not reported.

	REACT study (Randomized Evaluation of Assertive Community Treatment) (UK)
Author, Year (Country):	**Killaspy 2006[58]**
Results:	Committed suicide: ACT=0.8% (1/124) vs CMH=2.5% (3/119); between-groups comparison not reported Deliberate self-harm: ACT=8% (10/91) vs CMH=11% (13/75); mean difference= 0.72; P=0.40
Author, Year (Country):	**King 2006[57] (US)**
Population:	All adolescents who were psychiatrically hospitalized at a university-based or private hospital between August 1998 and December 2000.
Intervention 1:	Treatment as usual (TAU) varied and consisted of psychotherapy (100%), psychoactive medication (96.8%), alcohol/drug treatment (13.4%), partial hospitalization (18.0%), and community services (8.5%).
Intervention 2:	TAU plus Youth-Nominated Support Team – Version 1 (YST-1) consisted of youth nominating support persons from available caring others in their lives (including school, neighborhood/community, and family); support persons underwent training (psychoeducation sessions approximately 1.5-2hrs long), maintained weekly supportive contact with youth, and were contacted regularly by intervention specialists (mental health professionals with previous clinical experience with the youth). The psychoeducation included information on youth's treatment plan, risk factors for suicidal behavior, availability of emergency services, and strategies for communicating with adolescents.
Setting:	Not specified; 6 month follow-up period post hospitalization
N:	236; TAU=123, TAU+YST-1=113
Mean age, % female, race (variance):	Mean age = 12.0 (SD=3.3); TAU=11.9 (SD=3.5), TAU+YST-1=12.1 (SD=3.0) % female=68.2; TAU=67.4, TAU+YST-1=68.9 % White=82.4; TAU=79.6, TAU+YST-1=85.0
Outcome assessment:	Suicide attempts were measured through self-report on the Spectrum of Suicide Behavior Scale (Pfeffer, 1986)
Results:	No significant differences between groups in percent of adolescents with one or more suicide attempts % with 1 or more suicide attempts during the 6 month follow-up: TAU=11.7, TAU+YST-1=18.1% (fishers exact test, P=.22)
Author, Year (Country):	**King 2009[56] (US)**
Population:	All adolescents (aged 13-17) psychiatrically hospitalized in either a university or private hospital between 2002 and 2005.
Intervention 1:	Treatment as Usual (TAU) consisted of psychotherapy (mean # sessions=22.47), psychoactive medication (mean # different medications=1.66), medication follow-up (mean #=8.47), alcohol/drug treatment (n=4), psychiatric hospitalization (n=13), residential treatment (n=6)
Intervention 2:	Treatment as Usual plus Youth Support Team-II (TAU+YST-II) consisted of youth nominating caring adults from family, school, or neighborhood/community to serve as their supportive contacts. Intervention specialists were mental health professionals, assisted with the nomination process, and conducted psychoeducation sessions with the support persons. The psychoeducation included information on youth's treatment plan, risk factors for suicidal behavior, availability of emergency services, and strategies for communicating with adolescents. Support persons had weekly contact with the youth.
Setting:	Not specified; 12 month follow-up period post hospitalization
N:	346; TAU=171, TAU+YST-II=175 (N's reported and included in analysis after 12 month follow-up period)
Mean age, % female, race (variance):	Mean age=15.59 (SD=1.31), TAU=15.61 (SD=1.37), TAU+YST-II=15.56 (SD=1.24) % female=71 (same in both groups) % White=83.4, TAU=84, TAU+YST-II=83
Outcome assessment:	Presence or absence of one or more suicide attempts during follow-up was assessed via self-report, using the question, "Have you tried to kill yourself?" from the NIMH DISC-IV Mood Disorders Module.
Results:	No significant differences were found between groups for percent of adolescents with one or more attempts. % with one or more attempts in the 12 month follow-up period: TAU=35, TAU+YST-II=29, Chi-square (1, N=354)=0.66, p=.42 One suicide death occurred in the TAU group, no suicide deaths in the TAU+YST-II group

128

APPENDIX Y. RISK OF BIAS RATINGS FOR PRIMARY STUDIES RELATED TO REFERRAL/FOLLOW-UP SERVICES

Author Year	Sequence Generation		Allocation concealment		Blinding of participants, personnel, and outcome assessors		Incomplete outcome data		Selective outcome reporting		Other sources of bias		OVERALL risk of bias for the study as a whole
	Describe method	Was it adequate? Yes/No/Unclear	Describe method	Was it adequate? Yes/No/Unclear	Describe all measures used, if any, to blind study participants and personnel from knowledge of which intervention a participant received. Provide any information relating to whether intended blinding was effective.	Was knowledge of allocated intervention adequately prevented during the study? Yes/No/Unclear	Describe completeness of outcome data for each main outcome, including attrition and exclusions from analysis. State whether attrition and exclusions were reported, numbers in each intervention group (compared with total randomized participants), reasons for attrition/exclusions where reported, and any re-inclusions in analyses performed by review authors.	Were incomplete outcome data adequately addressed? Yes/No/Unclear	State how the possibility of selective outcome reporting was examined by review authors, and what was found.	Are reports of study free of suggestion of selective outcome reporting? Yes/No/Unclear	State any important concerns about bias not addressed in the tool. If particular questions/entries were pre-specified in the review's protocol, responses should be provided for each question/entry.	Was the study apparently free of other problems that could put it at a high risk of bias? Yes/No/Unclear	Low/ Unclear/ High
Beau-trais 2010[53]	Computer-generated random numbers.	Yes	Randomized by research staff who were not involved in the recruitment or clinical care of participants.	Yes	Psychiatric emergency service clinicians masked to allocation; allocation status not conveyed to clinical or data-collection staff.	Yes	327/327 analyzed; ITT.	Yes	No omissions of any expected suicide-related outcomes.	Yes	At baseline, number of prior attendances for self-harm was lower in the intervention group (P<0.07).	No	Unclear
Carter 2005[54]	Pregenerated randomization schedule.	Unclear	To maintain blinding to allocated group during recruitment, randomization was not revealed until after all information was entered and eligibility had been determined.	Yes	Clinical and research staff were blinded to allocation.	Yes	Well-described ITT analysis and pre-treatment group comparisons included in the article. Attritions and exclusions adequately documented and subject flowchart included in article. All 772 randomized were followed up. 76/378 randomized to treatment group did not consent to the intervention.	Yes	No omissions of any expected suicide-related outcomes.	Yes	20 participants in the control group received the intervention due to clerical errors but were included in the control group for the ITT analyses.	Unclear	Unclear
Gallo 2007[59]	Matched pairs randomized by coin flip.	Yes	Coin flip randomization done at the clinical practice level, so no allocation concealment related to patients was needed.	Yes	No information provided.	Unclear	Attritions and exclusions adequately documented. 12/650 (2%) excluded due to insufficient baseline data; vital statistics available on others.	Yes	No omissions of any expected suicide-related outcomes; authors state that outcome reporting and secondary data analysis were guided by cited standards. Prespecified study hypothesis was that risk of death would be reduced by the intervention.	Yes	Suicidal ideation higher in patients in intervention group at baseline.	Unclear	Unclear

Author Year	Sequence Generation		Allocation concealment		Blinding of participants, personnel, and outcome assessors		Incomplete outcome data		Selective outcome reporting		Other sources of bias		OVERALL risk of bias for the study as a whole
	Describe method	Was it adequate? Yes/No/Unclear	Describe method	Was it adequate? Yes/No/Unclear	Describe all measures used, if any, to blind study participants and personnel from knowledge of which intervention a participant received. Provide any information relating to whether intended blinding was effective.	Was knowledge of allocated intervention adequately prevented during the study? Yes/No/Unclear	Describe completeness of outcome data for each main outcome, including attrition and exclusions from analysis. State whether attrition and exclusions were reported, numbers in each intervention group (compared with total randomized participants), reasons for attrition/exclusions where reported, and any re-inclusions in analyses performed by review authors.	Were incomplete outcome data adequately addressed? Yes/No/Unclear	State how the possibility of selective outcome reporting was examined by review authors, and what was found.	Are reports of study free of suggestion of selective outcome reporting? Yes/No/Unclear	State any important concerns about bias not addressed in the other domains in the tool. If particular questions/entries were pre-specified in the review's protocol, responses should be provided for each question/entry.	Was the study apparently free of other problems that could put it at a high risk of bias? Yes/No/Unclear	Low/Unclear/High
Killaspy 2006[58]	No information provided other than a statement that treatment was randomized.	Unclear	Interviewer contacted administrator at trial center, who opened the appropriate numbered envelope giving details of the outcome of randomization.	Yes	No information provided.	Unclear	Attritions and exclusions adequately documented. Hospital admission data available for 243/251 at 18 months (97%); 68% response rate for interview at 18 months.	Yes	No omissions of any expected suicide-related outcomes.	Yes	The study appears to be free of other sources of bias.	Yes	Unclear
King 2006[57]	Random numbers table (even/odd assignment).	Yes	No allocation concealment.	No	"Raters were not blind to group status."	No	Well-described ITT analysis and pre-treatment group comparisons included in the article. Attritions and exclusions adequately documented and subject flowchart included in article.	Yes	No omissions of any expected suicide-related outcomes.	Yes	Differences among groups who met actually treated criteria and others in age, and family income (but not prior suicide attempts).	Unclear	Unclear
King 2009[56]	"Computerized balanced allocation strategy."	Yes	"Group assignments were unknown until the project manager generated them at the randomization website following the consent process (sequence unknown)."	Yes	"Independent evaluators were blinded to group assignment." No information on patient or provider blinding, though it would seem impossible given study design.	Assessors yes, participants unclear	Well-described ITT analysis and pre-treatment group comparisons included in the article. Attritions and exclusions adequately documented and subject flowchart included in article.	Yes	No omissions of any expected suicide-related outcomes.	Yes	The study appears to be free of other sources of bias.	Yes	Unclear

APPENDIX Z. STRENGTH OF EVIDENCE RATINGS FOR PRIMARY STUDIES RELATED TO REFERRAL/FOLLOW-UP SERVICES[a]

Table 1: Assertive Community Treatment

| Number of studies; # of subjects | Domains pertaining to strength of evidence | | | | Magnitude of effect | Strength of evidence |
	Risk of bias (Design/ Quality)	Consistency	Directness	Precision	Summary effect size (95% CI)	High, Moderate, Low, Insufficient
Assertive Community Treatment versus Community Mental Healthcare (Killaspy 2006)[58]						
Suicide deaths						
1; N=251	Medium (RCT/Unclear)	N/A	Indirect	Imprecise	0.8% vs 2.5%, *P* NR	Low
Deliberate self-harm						
1; N=251	Medium (RCT/Unclear)	N/A	Indirect	Imprecise	8% vs 11%; *P*=0.40	Low

Table 2: Case Management/Care Coordination

| Number of studies; # of subjects | Domains pertaining to strength of evidence | | | | Magnitude of effect | Strength of evidence |
	Risk of bias (Design/ Quality)	Consistency	Directness	Precision	Summary effect size (95% CI)	High, Moderate, Low, Insufficient
Depression Care Management versus Usual Care (Gallo 2007, Bogner 2007, Raue 2010; Prevention of Suicide in Primary Care Elderly: Collaborative Trial [PROSPECT])[59, 128, 129]						
Suicide deaths, n/1000 person-years (95% CI)						
1; N=599	Medium (RCT/Unclear)	N/A	Indirect	Imprecise	0.7 (0.0 to 4.2) vs UC=0, 0.0 (0.0 to 3.3)	Low

Table 3: Emergency contact "green" card

| Number of studies; # of subjects | Domains pertaining to strength of evidence | | | | Magnitude of effect | Strength of evidence |
	Risk of bias (Design/ Quality)	Consistency	Directness	Precision	Summary effect size (95% CI)	High, Moderate, Low, Insufficient
Emergency contact "green" card versus Standard Care (Morgan 1993 as cited in Mann 2005)[10]							
Suicide attempts						
1; not reported	Medium (RCT/Unclear)	N/A	Indirect	N/A	Not reported	Insufficient to Low

Table 4: Postcard/Mailing Interventions

Number of studies; # of subjects	Domains pertaining to strength of evidence					Magnitude of effect	Strength of evidence
	Risk of bias (Design/ Quality)	Consistency	Directness	Precision		Summary effect size (95% CI)	High, Moderate, Low, Insufficient
Postcard Intervention versus treatment as usual (Carter 2005/2007, Beautrais 2010)[53-55]							
Proportion of patients with repeat deliberate self poisoning at 12 months and 24 months (Carter 2005/2007)[54, 55]							
1; N=772	Medium (RCT/Unclear)	N/A	Indirect	Imprecise		12 months: 15.1% vs 17.3%; -2% (95% CI, -7% to 3%) 24 months: 21.2% vs 22.8%; -1.7% (95% CI, -7.5 to 4.2	Low
Cumulative number of repeat episodes of deliberate self poisoning at 12 months and 24 months (Carter 2005/2007)[54, 55]							
1; N=772	Medium (RCT/Unclear)	N/A	Indirect	Imprecise		12 months: IRR 0.55 (95% CI, 0.35 to 0.87) 24 months: 0.49 (95% CI, 0.33 to 0.73)	Low
Total proportions of patients re-presenting for self-harm at 12 months (Beautrais 2010)[53]							
1; N=327	Medium (RCT/Unclear)	N/A	Indirect	Imprecise		Adjusted OR=0.97 (95% CI, 0.58 to 1.62)	Low
Total number of self-harm re-presentations at 12 months (Beautrais 2010)[53]							
1; N=327	Medium (RCT/Unclear)	N/A	Indirect	Imprecise		Adjusted IRR=1.07 (95% CI, 0.80 to 1.43	Low
Regular Mailings vs Standard Care (Motto 2001 as cited in Mann 2005)[10]							
Suicide attempts							
1; not reported	Medium (RCT/Unclear)	N/A	Indirect	N/A		Not reported	Insufficient to Low

Table 5: Youth-Nominated Support Team (YST) plus Treatment As Usual

Number of studies; # of subjects	Domains pertaining to strength of evidence					Magnitude of effect	Strength of evidence
	Risk of rias (Design/ Quality)	Consistency	Directness	Precision		Summary effect size (95% CI)	High, Moderate, Low, Insufficient
Youth-Nominated Support Team (YST) plus Treatment As Usual versus Treatment As Usual (King 2006, King 2009)[56, 57]							
Suicide deaths							
1; N=448	Medium (RCT/Unclear)	N/A	Indirect	Imprecise		0.4% vs 0, P NR	Low
Proportion of adolescents with one or more suicide attempts							
2; N=737	Medium (RCT/Unclear)	Inconsistent	Indirect	Imprecise		YST-1: 17.3% vs 11.6%, $P=0.26$ YST-2: 13% vs 15%, $P=0.51$	Low

[a] This review did not evaluate any outcomes other than suicidal self-directed violence, and therefore no additional data on potential harms and side effects was investigated. Potential harms and side effects should always be considered when evaluating the strength of evidence and considering adoption of an intervention or referral/follow-up service.

APPENDIX AA. PEER REVIEW COMMENTS/AUTHOR RESPONSES

Reviewer	Comment	Response
Question 1:	**Are the objectives, scope, and methods for this review clearly described?**	
1	No. There was no discussion of the methods used for evaluating the strength of the evidence in a publication for drawing inferences about suicide prevention. There was a "boiler plate" discussion of the methods used for rating evidence. However, the draft did not provide adequate information about the way that this was applied for evaluating the strength of a paper for drawing inferences about suicide as an outcome, rather than for the primary outcome. More specifically, the literature reviewed included a number of papers reporting on studies conducted to evaluate treatments for other conditions or other outcomes (e.g., antidepressants for depression, or other interventions for suicidal ideation). Apparently, these were included because the papers included finding on suicide or suicide attempts, even though the studies were not designed to test hypotheses regarding suicide-related outcomes. There is a clear need to separate evaluations of the quality of the research as designed to test the primary hypotheses from the quality of the same studies for drawing inferences about suicide-related outcomes. The draft should have included information about methods for evaluating the quality of the studies for contributing to the literature on suicide. The absence of this information is a serious drawback.	We added a table to the final report which now provides this information to readers. This table also lists sample sizes for the various studies so readers can see how sample size compares for studies with different primary outcomes (i.e., those studies designed to prevent suicide versus studies in which this was not a primary or pre-specified outcome of interest).
1	As a related issue, the draft did not include a clear discussion of statistical power. Based on the discussion that was provided, statistical power did not appear to be included in the rates of the quality of research and the strength of the evidence. The methods section of the draft should have included a discussion of sample sizes and power, specifically for suicide prevention.	We discuss this issue throughout many of the sections of the report (e.g., stating "The majority of trials did not involve the necessary sample sizes (mean, 284.4 patients; standard deviation, 177.8) or follow-up durations (median, 8 weeks; range, 4 weeks to 2.5 years) required to adequately evaluate risk of suicide attempts or suicides. Therefore, these trials generally provided inadequate to low-strength evidence for drawing conclusions about risk of suicide attempts and suicides." in the section on pharmacotherapy. We also include a specific discussion of this issue pertaining to the table referenced in the above comment.
2	Yes. The objectives and scope are clearly described. Methods are clearly articulated and documentation re: process is provided. The authors state that the goal is to update work by reviewing literature that was not reviewed by Gaynes et al or Mann et al. It may be helpful for the reader to know the main findings from these reviews. The authors may also want to provide more detail about further support or lack thereof for Gaynes et al and Mann et als' assertions based on this review. Some of this is provided later in the document – but seems to be missing from the beginning of the review and is not consistently presented throughout.	We have updated the report to include more information on results from the Mann et al. (2005), Gaynes et al. (2004) and NICE (2011) systematic reviews throughout the report, and this information is also presented in tabular format.
3	Yes; no comment.	
4	Yes; no comment.	
5	No. Overall I think this is very well written. The objectives, scope and methods are fairly well described, but I do have several comments:	Thank you. Noted.
5	1. In the Key Questions 3 and 4 themselves, it needs to be made clearer what referral and follow-up services are. How are these approaches not subsumed under KQs 1 and 2—if they are a subset of the interventions covered in KQ 1 and 2, why are they being looked at separately? How is some change in referral or follow-up process not an intervention?—this needs to be clarified for Exec Summary and in introduction. Perhaps general access to mental health care may be a better/clearer construct than referral and follow-up??	We have clarified differences between studies cited in the "psychotherapy" versus "referral/follow-up services" sections of the report, which describes why these studies were discussed in two different sections when the treatments were similar.

Reviewer	Comment	Response
5	2. There are a few places where there may be inconsistencies in the terminology used, and the terminology may not be consistent with the new VA DOD terminology for self harm behaviors. I would overtly acknowledge and reference this new nomenclature early on, include a table on it, and make sure that it is consistent throughout the document.	We added a description and definition of "suicidal self-directed violence," the adopted VA/DoD nomenclature, in both the executive summary and the introduction section of the report. We have also updated the report with consistent terminology throughout.
5	3. Because this follows up on previous reviews, I think it would be important to include some type of summary at the end of the response to each KQ that incorporates or acknowledges the previous relevant findings from those reviews. For several of the KQs, you do not have findings, but perhaps that is because you are only reviewing what was published between 2005 and 2011. Perhaps there are older findings that would provide more information or context for your findings. The findings from the previous reviews also should be addressed/integrated into the Discussion/Summary section so the reader can see if and how (or not) things may have changed.	We have updated the report to include more information on results from the Mann et al. (2005), Gaynes et al. (2004) and NICE (2011) systematic reviews throughout the report, and this information is also presented in tabular format.
5	4. In the Exec Summ response to KQ2, the response is written as if suicide is the main or perhaps only outcome of interest. But you are also looking at other suicide behavior outcomes such as suicide attempts. In some places, like on page 3 and on page 15 this is not clear.	We have made these corrections and updated the report to consistently use the term suicidal self-directed violence in reference to outcomes.
5	5. doing this review again so soon—have there been a lot of new studies/what is rationale? Who was the proponent for this review—can that be listed?	We have updated the methods section to more clearly describe the rationale and request for the report.
5	6. In the Exec Summary it is striking to me that 16,502 papers were initially reviewed-these are all since 2005? Do you want to briefly describe your key or main inclusion criteria (I focus a lot on Exec Summary because this is all many readers will actually read.	We have added this brief description to the executive summary.
6	Yes. The questions appear sound, but an explanation of what "suicidal self-directed violence" means would be helpful.	We have defined and cited this terminology.
7	Yes; no comment.	
8	Yes. The objectives, scope and methods are clear. I think the focus on RCTs is key as these studies have greater internal validity, and many other syntheses have made the choice to combine RCTs with observational studies. Keeping the focus on RCTs makes it clear how few high-quality data are available regarding preventative interventions for suicide, particularly in Veteran and military populations.	Thank you. Noted, and we agree that the focus on RCTs helps limit the report to the highest quality research available on suicidal self-directed violence outcomes.
8	Since this review explicitly uses the Mann review as a starting point, I would recommend that the synthesis build even more upon the Mann review. (The report already does do this, in part, in the more detailed sections.) Specifically I would recommend acknowledging where there is sufficient evidence to confirm the conclusions of this prior synthesis, where there is insufficient new evidence to comment on prior conclusions, and where there is sufficient new evidence that conflicts with prior conclusions. This should be done in addition to findings from the recent literature in new areas of intervention. At this point, there are several statements emphasizing contrasts to the Mann report which seem more a function of insufficient new evidence rather than new evidence that conflicts with prior conclusions. (For example, no new literature on clozapine was reviewed and there are insufficient data from studies of other antipsychotics to make a statement about other antipsychotic medications or the group of antipsychotic medications.) Insufficient new evidence would not seem to overturn prior findings, unless there was further synthesis of both the older and the newer findings.	We have updated the report to include more information on results from the Mann et al. (2005), Gaynes et al. (2004) and NICE (2011) systematic reviews throughout the report, and this information is also presented in tabular format.
8	I would also recommend mentioning the Bagley VA Evidence Based Synthesis earlier on as he and his colleagues also reviewed literature on psychotherapy and pharmacotherapy in addition to larger public health interventions.	We have included information about this report and scope differences in the methods section of both the executive summary and the body of the report.

Reviewer	Comment	Response
8	On a minor note, this review started with studies published as of January 2005 and the Mann review covered until June 2005. Thus there is some overlap in the dates covered in the two reviews. Given review inclusion criteria, this results in an important 2005 publication being included in the Mann report (Brown, JAMA 2005) and not this report. Knowledgeable readers will likely be looking for this paper.	We clarified that articles included in this report are only those not previously included in the Mann et al. report, and hence articles such as the Brown (2005) paper were excluded (pages 1 and 9).
2.	**Is there any indication of bias in our synthesis of the evidence?**	
1	Possible. I used what I viewed as potentially positive findings that were published during the relevant period as markers for evaluating the draft. One was the Lauterbach study discussed in my response to question 3. This was a report of a study designed to determine whether adjunctive lithium prevented suicide reattempts in patients with depression or bipolar disorder who survived and initial attempt. Unfortunately, the investigators were unable to achieve the planned sample size. However, a finding based on post-hoc analyses suggested that lithium may have reduced deaths from suicide. I would have been interested in seeing how the draft evaluated this claim. However, the article was not included.	Noted. As you state, this article was not included. This is because the study was conducted in Germany, a country outside the scope of this review, per initial scoping agreement with the stakeholders/CPG group requesting the report.
1	Another was the Hatcher article on the effect of problem-solving therapy for suicide prevention. The article reports that there was no significant effect of problem-solving therapy in the entire sample. However, they report that a planned subgroup analysis demonstrated that the intervention was effective in the subsample of the subjects who had survived a suicide attempt prior to the index attempt that led to study entry. The article was included in the review but the planned subgroup analysis was not mentioned.	We have updated this section, making specific reference to these findings.
1	The two articles I mentioned represent two of the most significant potential advances of the past few years. Personally, I was looking to the Evidence Synthesis for guidance about the evaluation of the reported findings. However, neither of the salient findings were addressed. It is possible that this reflects poor implementation. However, it is also possible that this may reflect a bias towards negative findings.	Noted. We have attempted to use the most current, objective, and stringent methods for preventing bias in this report, and have addressed the comments about these two studies above.
2	No; No.	Noted.
3	No; no comment.	
4	No; no comment.	
5	No; no comment.	
6	Yes; no comment.	
7	No; no comment.	
8	No. The study selection criteria, quality assessment criteria, and rating of the strength of the evidence are clearly described. I agree with the focus on RCTs, given the limitations of the evidence from other study designs.	Thank you. Noted, and we agree that the focus on RCTs helps limit the report to the highest quality research available on suicidal self-directed violence outcomes.
8	Please include a table for 317 studies and reasons for exclusion.	Appendix W is a table of excluded studies, and contains information on reasons for exclusion.
3.	**Are there any _published_ or _unpublished_ studies that we may have overlooked?**	
1	Yes, I used what I viewed as important papers published during the relevant period as markers to evaluate the literature that was reviewed. Specifically, I searched for, "Lauterbach E. Felber W. Muller-Oerlinghausen B. Ahrentos B. Bronisch T, et al Adjunctive lithium treatment in the prevention of suicidal behaviour in depressive disorders: a randomised, placebo-controlled, 1-year trial. Acta Psychiatrica Scandinavica. 118(6):469-79, 2008". Its absence from the literature that was identified raises serious questions about the process for identifying relevant literature.	Noted. As you state, this article was not included. This is because the study was conducted in Germany, a country outside the scope of this review, per initial scoping agreement with the stakeholders/CPG group requesting the report. We have, however, included this article in a non-systematic addition to the review, per your suggestion. This information is now contained within the pharmacotherapy section of the report.

Reviewer	Comment	Response
1	In addition, I have heard verbal reports that findings were available, but not yet published, from a second study of cognitive behavioral therapy for suicide prevention in attempt survivors to determine whether it decreased the rate of reattempts. I may be useful to contact Dr. Gregory Brown from the University of Pennsylvania (gregbrow@mail.med.upenn.edu) to get more information.	Noted. Per follow-up discussions with the CPG and stakeholders, the decision was made not to include unpublished studies or data analysis in this report.
2	Yes. A. In terms of intervention, several key studies seem to have been left out of the psychotherapy results section- perhaps because they were published prior or after – this makes it seem like even less work has been down in this area. See comment 1A above.	Noted; see responses below for each study.
2	1: Brown GK, Ten Have T, Henriques GR, Xie SX, Hollander JE, Beck AT. Cognitive therapy for the prevention of suicide attempts: a randomized controlled trial. JAMA. 2005 Aug 3;294(5):563-70. PubMed PMID: 16077050.	Though our search did, indeed, capture this article, we did not include it because of its inclusion in the previously published Mann et al. (2005) report. We note this exclusion criterion in the report on pages 1 and 9.
2	2: Bruce ML, Ten Have TR, Reynolds CF 3rd, Katz II, Schulberg HC, Mulsant BH, Brown GK, McAvay GJ, Pearson JL, Alexopoulos GS. Reducing suicidal ideation and depressive symptoms in depressed older primary care patients: a randomized controlled trial. JAMA. 2004 Mar 3;291(9):1081-91. PubMed PMID: 14996777.	This study was published prior to the beginning of our search dates, and was therefore not included in the report. Information published prior to June, 2005 was addressed in the Mann et al. (2005) report, and so as to avoid duplication, we did not include any such studies in this current review.
2	1: Simpson GK, Tate RL, Whiting DL, Cotter RE. Suicide prevention after traumatic brain injury: a randomized controlled trial of a program for the psychological treatment of hopelessness. J Head Trauma Rehabil. 2011 Jul-Aug;26(4):290-300. PubMed PMID: 21734512.	This study did not include reports on outcomes included in this report (i.e., suicide and suicidal self-directed violence); therefore it was excluded from the review.
2	B. For TBI among veterans may want to include Brenner LA, Ignacio RV, Blow FC. Suicide and traumatic brain injury among individuals seeking Veterans Health Administration services. J Head Trauma Rehabil. 2011 Jul-Aug;26(4):257-64. PubMed PMID: 21734509	This study is not a RCT and was therefore excluded from the review; however, this study was considered for the companion review conducted by our research team on suicide risk and assessment.
3	No; At least none that I am aware of	Noted.
4	No; no comment.	
5	No; Not that I know of	Noted.
6	No; no comment.	
7	No; no comment.	
8	I am not aware of any additional RCTs in this area during this time frame.	Noted.
4.	**Please write additional suggestions or comments below. If applicable, please indicate the page and line numbers from the draft report.**	
1	The Mann article reviewed articles through June, 2005. Please provide more specifics about how you ensured that there were neither gaps, nor overlaps with the Mann article.	We clarified that articles included in this report are only those not previously included in the Mann et al. report, and hence articles such as the Brown (2005) paper were excluded (pages 1 and 9).
1	The methods suggest that the review process did not distinguish articles on the basis of the goals or the aims of the research that was reported. This is important. Research that was conducted, for example, to determine whether a specific intervention led to reductions in suicidal ideation, may have been well designed and adequately powered to address that question. However, even if it reported on the number of subjects who attempted or died from suicide, it would probably be underpowered to address these outcomes. This distinction should be considered in evaluating the quality of the studies reviewed.	We added a table to the final report which now provides this information to readers. This table also lists sample sizes for the various studies so readers can see how sample size compares for studies with different primary outcomes (i.e., those studies designed to prevent suicide versus studies in which this was not a primary or pre-specified outcome of interest).

Reviewer	Comment	Response
1	The first sentence under "Pharmacotherapy results" states, "Studies evaluated antidepressants .... For their efficacy in prevention of suicide .... " In fact, none of the studies were designed or intended to evaluate efficacy for suicide prevention. The sentence is incorrect.	We have updated the sentence to read: Studies evaluated antidepressants, atypical antipsychotics, mood stabilizers, and omega-3 supplements and reported their efficacy in prevention of suicidal self-directed violence in non-Veteran/military populations.
1	The first paragraph under "Pharmacotherapy results" states that 9 studies were reviewed, then it cites 10. This should be clarified.	We have clarified that these were 9 studies published in 10 publications.
1	Among the citations in the first paragraph under Pharmacology results,the citations numbered 15-20 and 24 were conducted to evaluate depression as an outcome. They were not designed or powered for suicide-related outcomes. This should be stated.	See above comment re: providing this information in tabular format.
1	The conclusions stated at the end of the first paragraph refer only to suicide as an outcome. This is inconsistent with the definition of the scope of the review that addresses "suicidal self-directed violence." As written, the conclusions are confusing and misleading.	This sentence has been updated to read: "Therefore, they are felt to be of low strength, and are insufficient for determining the effectiveness of various combinations of antidepressant medications for reducing suicidal self-directed violence."
1	The reports cited as 21 and 22 were written to report on outcomes related to suicidal ideation. This should be acknowledged.	See above comment re: providing this information in tabular format.
1	The report cited as 23 included suggestive, apparently post-hoc, analyses of greater self-harm with certain medications. It may be misleading to conclude only that it said nothing about deaths from suicide.	Added results of subgroup analyses showing increased risk in patients taking venlafaxine vs SSRIs and those taking benzodiazepines.
1	Studies cited as 25-27 in the second paragraph were not conducted to evaluate the effectiveness of antipsychotic medications in reducing suicide deaths. This should be acknowledged.	See above comment re: providing this information in tabular format.
1	The point of reference 28 was that there were no drug related increases in suicidal ideation as an adverse drug effect. It should be acknowledged that the study was not conducted to test for decreases in death from suicide.	See above comment re: providing this information in tabular format.
1	The last sentence of the second paragraph say there is a contrast between the cited papers and findings of an effect of clozapine. In fact, the findings on clozapine reflect a difference between that medication and another atypical antipsychotic. There is no contrast.	This sentence has been updated to read: "Notably, the previous review by Mann and colleagues reported an antisuicidal effect of clozapine, an atypical antipsychotic medication."
1	The text in the first sentence of the third paragraph is incorrect. Reference 29 was a 2.5 year study. Reference 30 was an 8 week study.	This correction has been made.
1	Reference 29 found no significant differences between lithium and valproate, but it is not correct to say that it did not have suicide or suicide attempt outcomes.	This has been clarified in the report.
1	Reference 30 focused on ideation and related symptoms; this should be acknowledged.	We did not include ideation as an outcome in this report, and therefore those results are not reported. However, we do report primary outcome information from studies in tabular format.
1	The reference for citation 31 is incomplete. It is from the British Journal of Psychiatry.	This correction has been made.
1	The review should acknowledge that 31 was intended to report on outcomes related to ideation and related measures rather than attempts or deaths from suicide.	We did not include ideation as an outcome in this report, and therefore those results are not reported. However, we do report primary outcome information from studies in tabular format.
1	Reference 32 reported that problem solving was effective for decreasing repeated self-harm in a subsample of patients with multiple previous episodes. This should be acknowledged.	See above comment re: the Hatcher paper.
1	Citation 39 referred to a study evaluating 64 adults with history of self harm. It may have reported on deaths,but it was conducted primarily to look at other outcomes.	See above comment re: providing this information in tabular format.

Reviewer	Comment	Response
1	Citation 45 reported a decreases in ideation. This should be acknowledged. In its critique, it is not clear what was meant by the phrase "had methods that suggested an unclear risk of bias."	We did not report ideation outcomes in this report. The latter sentence has been clarified to read: "...used methods resulting in an unclear risk of bias."
1	Citation 52 is a secondary analyses of a study of an intervention similar to that reported in 45. It should be acknowledged that the outcome of interest was total mortality, not suicide. The study was conducted to test for decreases in suicidal ideation. Moreover, it is not clear why 52 is discussed in a section separate from 45 when the interventions were so similar	See above comment re: providing outcome information in tabular format. We have clarified differences between studies cited in the "psychotherapy" versus "referral/follow-up services" sections of the report, which describes why these studies were discussed in two different sections when the treatments were similar.
2	A. Page 1 – 20% of veterans – believe this number originally came from the work of Kaplan et al. It is somewhat problematic in that Veteran was broadly defined and likely included other cohorts (e.g. active duty).	This data came from NVDRS, which does include anyone who has served in the armed forces. We have modified this sentence to be more clear about who the 20% represent.
2	B. Recent research has focused more on warning signs vs. risk factors as a prevention strategy. May want to consider including this. May also want to include warning signs in Analytic Model. 1: Rudd MD, Berman AL, Joiner TE Jr, Nock MK, Silverman MM, Mandrusiak M, Van Orden K, Witte T. Warning signs for suicide: theory, research, and clinical applications. Suicide Life Threat Behav. 2006 Jun;36(3):255-62. Review. PubMed PMID: 16805653.	Any intervention RCTs meeting inclusion criteria were included in this report, and a separate report completed by our research team is addressing risk factors and warning signs. We have included both risk factor and warning sign terminology in the analytical model.
2	C. A number of studies are currently underway in the VA – this seems worth mentioning – information could be found on clinical trials.gov or VA websites.	We have included this information in the discussion.
2	D. As Analytic model 1 and 2 appear to be identical may way to combine.	We agree, and have combined the analytical models as you suggest.
3	This is an excellent review of RCTs to date and is an important followup to the Mann review. Essentially it states that we are a long way from where we would like to be in understanding what is and is not an effective intervention. As it pointed out, the base rate of suicide is so low, the phemenon itself so complex and the interventions so diverse that it is difficult to put together an RCT, particularly a blinded RCT, with sufficient power while appropriately limiting the variables being studied. This may account for the dearth of RCTs. In the end, it may be that other forms of evidence, albeit lower level evidence (e.g. aggregated performance improvement data), will be necessary to identify successful interventions.	Noted, and we agree. We have made this suggestion in the discussion section of the report.
4	None.	Noted.
5	In the executive summary, on page 1 I would include the reference number for the Gaynes review right after you write "Gaynes and colleagues", not at the end of the sentence.	We have made this change.
5	On page 3, you write about two studies on mood stabilizers that did not have any suicide or suicide attempt outcomes—if not, why were these included in the review?	We have clarified this sentence to read: "These trials reported no instances of suicidal self-directed violence for the duration of either study." The trials did collect information on these outcomes, though no such events occurred.
5	Intro section on pages 6 and 7 is nicely written	Noted. Dr. Denneson was responsible for much of this section.
5	In the inclusion criteria section you don't include the specific dates for including the studies you are reviewing (ie from 2005 to 2011)	We have made this addition.
5	The limitations section should also acknowledge that your search strategy specifically looked for keywords and terms related to suicide/suicide behaviors. There may have been potentially relevant manuscripts published about various interventions which did not have those terms attached to them. There may be a bit more to say about the limitations of the search strategy itself in the Limitations section	We have included this information in the appropriate sections.

Reviewer	Comment	Response
6	This is a very thorough review of suicide prevention interventions. The authors make a good case for focus on RCTs only and the four questions appear sound. I have a few suggestions for this report.	Noted.
6	First, it might be helpful to justify why other forms of violent death/ behavior were not included. There might be public health interventions that are relevant to suicide prevention that address other causes of death such as homicide, accidents, "suicide by cop" or accidental overdose.	We have included comments to this effect in the discussion section.
6	Second, more discussion on the heterogeneity of studies is warranted. Many of the RCTs reported might have had stringent exclusion criteria (as the authors noted that patient who are suicidal are often excluded from trials), often leading to minimal changes in outcome. Some recommendations on how such criteria should be modified would help in the development of more generalizable studies in the future.	We have added more information on this topic in the results and discussion sections of the report.
7	Page (i) wrong header	This correction has been made.
7	p. 3, p. 19 should be "usual care alone" rather than "along"	This correction has been made.
7	p. 5 Bruce et al 2004 is the primary reference for the PROSPECT study. Gallo et al was designed to examine all-cause mortality	Agreed; however, we report as the primary citation the article which reports on our outcome of interest (i.e., suicidal self-directed violence), and therefore we cite Gallo et al., whereas Bruce et al. is cited for inclusion as a companion article which was reviewed for methods information about the study. Similar examples are also cited as such in the report (e.g., the TADS trial papers).
7	p. 6 "suicide screen" is problematic language since suicide does not meet many clinical epidemiologic criteria for appropriate screening targets, nor is there an evidence base to commend a particular technique to assess suicidality	Noted. We have removed this terminology from the sentence.
7	p. 14 change from number of articles to number of publications is confusing	We agree that the paragraph can be confusing due to the fact that some studies are published in more than one paper. We hope the Literature Flow Chart can provide clarification.
8	For clarity in the narrative, it may help to group studies (e.g. those assessing psychotherapy) into those with sufficient sample size and duration to actually have a chance of addressing the outcomes of suicides and suicide attempts and those that do not. Currently the narrative is organized primarily around the specific psychotherapeutic intervention which often have been examined in only a single study with quality issues.	Though we did not group studies in this manner, we have added this information in tabular format to address this point, comparing sample size and commenting on statistical power in the studies.
8	Would recommend a short discussion section in the executive summary.	
5.	**Are there any clinical performance measures, programs, quality improvement measures, patient care services, or conferences that will be directly affected by this report? If so, please provide detail.**	
1	I am concerned that the quality of the draft report as it is currently written could represent a barrier to implementation of new advances. I do not think the report should be released in its current form.	Noted. The report was revised per reviewer feedback, and is released to the public after suggested changes have been made.
2	The lack of evidence-based treatments would be expected to impact care for suicidal veterans.	Yes, it could. It is our hope that future research will continue to inform evidence-based treatment research and implementation so that Veterans and members of the military may have access to effective, evidence-based care.
3	This report will be viewed with interest by many in Patient Care Services, particularly those involved in suicide prevention. I think that the report validates what many believe – that suicidal behavior is complex, difficult to predict and can be difficult to prevent.	Noted.
4	Not that I am aware of	Noted.
6	Office of Mental Health Operations, Canandaigua COE, National Center on Homelessness among Veterans, VA Cooperative Studies Program, local police	Noted.

Reviewer	Comment	Response
7	Suicide prevention coordinator programs	Noted.
8	In my reading of this summary, there were no RCTs at all for interventions for military populations or Veterans. There was insufficient evidence for specific pharmacotherapies or psychotherapies in general English speaking populations in eligible countries. The strongest evidence for psychotherapies was moderate evidence for no benefit of problem solving therapy for patients with suicide attempts. Therefore, this review suggests no evidence to support changes in or new clinical performance measures or mandated programs that emphasize these interventions for suicide prevention. The synthesis does outline an important research agenda for the VA.	Noted, and we agree that, in the case of an absence of evidence, particularly for the populations of interest, this report provides information related to areas of research in need of further investigation.
6.	**Please provide any recommendations on how this report can be revised to more directly address or assist implementation needs.**	
1	The organization of the report is generic, and as such, it does not appear to have been designed specifically to address suicide prevention. It may have been better to organize the report around the clinical ecology of suicide, where low numbers demand larger studies, and where information about surrogate endpoints (e.g., suicidal ideation) may be important, but where they may not translate directly into the prevention of suicide-related behaviors.	Though we did not group studies in this manner, we have added a table to address this point, comparing sample size and statistical power in the studies.
1	The evaluation and discussion should, perhaps, focus on studies that had adequate power to detect effects, and those where claims of effects were made. It should acknowledge that there may be promising findings regarding suicide ideation as an outcome, but that these were outside of the scope of the review. It should also be acknowledged that there were promising interventions, some that have been the subject of recent research, but where adequately powered clinical trials have not yet been conducted.	We have added a section on this topic, and included a table to present information on statistical power and primary outcomes in the trials. We have acknowledged that there may be promising findings regarding suicide ideation as an outcome, but that these were outside of the scope of the review as part of the discussion section.
2	A. Are there common elements of the most promising interventions that could be incorporated into current practice? May be helpful to review: **Oxford Text of Suicidology and Suicide Prevention, DOI: 10.1093/med/9780198570059.003.0058,** **Chapter 58 The psychological and behavioural treatment of suicidal behaviour** **What are the common elements of treatments that work?** M **David Rudd**, Ben Williams and **David** RM Trotter This chapter provides a review of all currently available clinical trials targeting suicidal behaviour. In contrast to some previous available reviews, the focus of the current chapter is on identifying **common elements** of treatments that work. More specifically, we attempted to answer the question, what do treatments that work have in com- mon? A number of psychological treatments have emerged as effective or potentially effective at reducing suicidal behaviour (i.e. **suicide** attempts). There now appear to be a number of identifiable core **elements** for treatments that have proven effective at reducing **suicide** attempts, all with direct and meaningful implications for day to day clinical practice. We also point out limitations in current sci- ence, including problematic follow-up periods and questions about the high-risk nature of some study samples.	We have reviewed this chapter, and agree that this non-systematic review could contain guidance for future research directions in the area of suicidal self- directed violence prevention interventions. We have added this citation to the discussion section.
2	B. A trial of the PST (Hatcher et al. 2011) among Veterans may be indicated – wonder if this recommendation should be made.	We have included a more in depth discussion of this trial in the results section, and have highlighted this trial in the discussion section.

Reviewer	Comment	Response
3	Related to the comments in #4. Suicide prevention efforts have been under way in VHA and DoD for a number of years. Many interventions have a great deal of face validity, and, for reasons already cited, it may be difficult to generate RCT data to test them in traditional ways. The report could be enlarged to include a section summarizing the efforts to date, along with population data spanning the last X number of years. It need not make any statements about any particular intervention, since doing so would not be consistent with the approach taken in this review.	We have now included more such information on earlier trials found in other systematic reviews such as Mann et al. (2005) and Gaynes et al. (2004) to provide a more comprehensive discussion of this point. Population data was included in the background sections, and will be covered in additional detail in a companion report by our research team on Suicide Risk and Assessment.
4	Given the findings, there is little to implement.	Noted.
5	As per above, would flesh out Exec Summary a bit more since this is what most people will read	We have expanded this section per your recommendations.
6	It would be helpful to shorten the executive summary into a one-page synopsis of the available evidence, what more needs to be researched, and from the available research, what is actionable for VA leaders to implement as public health, practice-based, or provider level interventions. For example, the Office of Mental Health Services uses a reporting tool in which key findings and progress updates are presented in tabular form.	We agree that a brief summary format is beneficial for some readers. In addition to the executive summary, we report findings in a "management brief" single page format which is electronically disseminated following the final report publication.
7	Less mechanical and repetitive approach to organizing the manuscript.	We have attempted to organize the report in a clear manner, consistent with standard systematic review reporting criteria.
8	Please see above. The evidence does not support immediate implementation of any suicide prevention program per se.	Noted.
7.	**Please provide us with contact details of any additional individuals/stakeholders who should be made aware of this report.**	
1	The report should be revised extensively before it is disseminated.	Noted. We have made revisions as recommended by the peer reviewers.
5	Jan Kemp, Ira Katz, Toni Zeiss from VA Office of Mental Health Services should just have a bit of a heads up	Thank you for these recommendations.
6	Jan Kemp and Rob Bossarte, Canandaigua COE/VACO; Ira Katz, MD, Office of Mental Health Operations/VACO. DOD	Thank you for these recommendations.
7	Jan Kemp	Thank you for these recommendations.
8	Drs. Zeiss, Kemp, Katz, Schohn in Central Office. VISN 19 MIRECC, VISN 2 Center of Excellence for Suicide Prevention, Defense Centers of Excellence for Psychological Health.	Thank you for these recommendations.

APPENDIX BB. ABBREVIATIONS

Abbreviation	Term
AHRQ	Agency for Healthcare Research and Quality
CAMS	Collaborative Assessment and Management of Suicidality
CBT	Cognitive Behavioral Therapy
CI	Confidence interval
DBT	Dialectical Behavior Therapy
DoD	Department of Defense
DSM	Diagnostic and Statistical Manual of Mental Disorders
EBPWG	Evidence Based Practice Working Group
E-CAU	Enhanced Care As Usual
EPC	Evidence-based Practice Center
GRADE	Grading of Recommendations Assessment, Development, and Evaluation
HR	Hazard ratio
IMPACT	Improving Mood: Promoting Access to Collaborative Treatment
IRR	Incident Risk Ratio
ITT	Intention-to-treat
LOCF	Last Observation Carried Forward
MBT	Mentalization Based Treatment
N	Sample size
N/A	Not applicable
NDI	National Death Index
NICE	National Institute for Health and Clinical Excellence
OR	Odds ratio
PROSPECT	Prevention of Suicide in Primary Care Elderly: Collaborative Trial
PSA	Public Service Announcement
RCT	Randomized controlled trial
REACT	Randomized Evaluation of Assertive Community Treatment
RR	Relative risk
SCM	Structured Clinical Management
SD	Standard deviation
SSRI	Selective Serotonin Reuptake Inhibitor
STEPPS	Systems Training for Emotional Predictability and Problem Solving
SUD	Substance Use Disorder
TADS	Treatment for Adolescents With Depression Study
TBI	Traumatic Brain Injury
TORDIA	Treatment of SSRI-Resistant Depression in Adolescents
UK	United Kingdom
US	United States
VA	Veterans Affairs
VHA	Veterans Health Administration
YST	Youth-Nominated Support Team

APPENDIX CC. EXCLUDED STUDIES

The following full-text publications were considered for inclusion but failed to meet the criteria for this report.

Exclusion codes:

1 = non-English language
2 = ineligible country
3 = ineligible outcome
4 = ineligible intervention
5 = did not evaluate interventions
6 = ineligible publication type
7 = ineligible systematic review due to limitations in quality
8 = ineligible nonsystematic regulatory agency analysis
9 = ineligible design

Excluded Trials	Exclusion Code
1 Agius M, Gardner J, Liu K, Zaman R. An audit to compare discharge rates and suicidality between antidepressant monotherapies prescribed for unipolar depression. Psychiatria Danubina. 2010;22(2):350-3.	3
2 Agius M, Shah S, Ramkisson R, Murphy S, Zaman R. Three year outcomes of an early intervention for psychosis service as compared with treatment as usual for first psychotic episodes in a standard community mental health team - final results. Psychiatr Danub. 2007 Sep;19(3):130-8.	9
3 Agomelatine: new drug. Adverse effects and no proven efficacy. Prescrire Int. 2009 Dec;18(104):241-5.	6
4 Aksoy-Poyraz C, Ozdemir A, Ozmen M, Arikan K, Ozkara C. Electroconvulsive therapy for bipolar depressive and mixed episode with high suicide risk after epilepsy surgery. Epilepsy & Behavior. 2008 Nov;13(4):707-9.	2
5 Alexander MJ, Haugland G, Ashenden P, Knight E, Brown I. Coping with thoughts of suicide: techniques used by consumers of mental health services. Psychiatr Serv. 2009 Sep;60(9):1214-21.	5
6 Alexopoulos GS, Katz IR, Bruce ML, et al. Remission in Depressed Geriatric Primary Care Patients: A Report From the PROSPECT Study. The American Journal of Psychiatry. 2005 Apr;162(4):718-24.	3
7 Andersson N, Ledogar RJ. The CIET Aboriginal Youth Resilience Studies: 14 Years of Capacity Building and Methods Development in Canada. Pimatisiwin. 2008 Summer;6(2):65-88.	6
8 Andrade C, Bhakta SG, Singh NM. Controversy revisited: Selective serotonin reuptake inhibitors in paediatric depression. World J Biol Psychiatry. 2006;7(4):251-60.	6
9 Angst J, Angst F, Gerber-Werder R, Gamma A. Suicide in 406 Mood-Disorder Patients With and Without Long-Term Medication: A 40 to 44 Years' Follow-Up. Archives of Suicide Research. 2005 Sep;9(3):279-300.	2
10 Apter A, Lipschitz A, Fong R, et al. Evaluation of suicidal thoughts and behaviors in children and adolescents taking paroxetine. J Child Adolesc Psychopharmacol. 2006 Feb-Apr;16(1-2):77-90.	6
11 Arkov K, Rosenbaum B, Christiansen L, Jonsson H, Munchow M. [Treatment of suicidal patients: The Collaborative Assessment and Management of Suicidality]. Ugeskr Laeger. 2008 Jan 14;170(3):149-53.	1

Excluded Trials	Exclusion Code
12 Army Suicide Prevention Task Force. Army Health Promotion, Risk Reduction and Suicide Prevention: Report 2010. Washington, D.C.: Department of Defense; 2010.	6
13 Arnevik E, Wilberg T, Urnes O, Johansen M, Monsen JT, Karterud S. Psychotherapy for personality disorders: short-term day hospital psychotherapy versus outpatient individual therapy - a randomized controlled study. Eur Psychiatry. 2009 Mar;24(2):71-8.	2
14 Asarnow JR, Porta G, Spirito A, et al. Suicide attempts and nonsuicidal self-injury in the treatment of resistant depression in adolescents: findings from the TORDIA study. J Am Acad Child Adolesc Psychiatry. 2011 Aug;50(8):772-81.	6
15 Aseltine RH, Jr., James A, Schilling EA, Glanovsky J. Evaluating the SOS suicide prevention program: a replication and extension. BMC Public Health. 2007;7:161.	9
16 Baber K, Bean G. Frameworks: A community-based approach to preventing youth suicide. Journal of Community Psychology. 2009 Aug;37(6):684-96.	3
17 Bajbouj M, Merkl A, Schlaepfer TE, et al. Two-year outcome of vagus nerve stimulation in treatment-resistant depression. J Clin Psychopharmacol. 2010 Jun;30(3):273-81.	2
18 Bakim B, Karamustafalioglu K, Akpinar A. Suicides and attempted suicides in alcohol and other substance use disorders. Bagimlik Dergisi. 2007 Aug;8(2):91-6.	1
19 Bakim B, Karamustafalioglu K, Ogutcen O, Yumrukcal H. Alcohol-Substance Use Disorders in HIV Infection. Bagimlik Dergisi. 2006 Aug;7(2):91-7.	1
20 Baldessarini RJ, Pompili M, Tondo L. Suicidal risk in antidepressant drug trials. Arch Gen Psychiatry. 2006 Mar;63(3):246-8.	6
21 Baldessarini RJ, Tondo L, Davis P, Pompili M, Goodwin FK, Hennen J. Decreased risk of suicides and attempts during long-term lithium treatment: a meta-analytic review. Bipolar Disord. 2006 Oct;8(5 Pt 2):625-39.	7
22 Baldwin DS, Reines EH, Guiton C, Weiller E. Escitalopram therapy for major depression and anxiety disorders. Ann Pharmacother. 2007 Oct;41(10):1583-92.	6
23 Balis T, Postolache TT. Ethnic differences in adolescent suicide in the United States. International Journal of Child Health and Human Development. 2008;1(3,Spec Iss):281-96.	6
24 Ballard ED, Pao M, Horowitz L, Lee LM, Henderson DK, Rosenstein DL. Aftermath of suicide in the hospital: institutional response. Psychosomatics. 2008 Nov-Dec;49(6):461-9.	6
25 Banerjee S, Hellier J, Dewey M, et al. Sertraline or mirtazapine for depression in dementia (HTA-SADD): a randomised, multicentre, double-blind, placebo-controlled trial. Lancet. 2011 Jul 30;378(9789):403-11.	3
26 Bangs ME, Tauscher-Wisniewski S, Polzer J, et al. Meta-analysis of suicide-related behavior events in patients treated with atomoxetine. Journal of the American Academy of Child & Adolescent Psychiatry. 2008 Feb;47(2):209-18.	6
27 Barak A. Emotional support and suicide prevention through the Internet: A field project report. Computers in Human Behavior. 2007 Mar;23(2):971-84.	2
28 Barak Y, Olmer A, Aizenberg D. Antidepressants reduce the risk of suicide among elderly depressed patients. Neuropsychopharmacology. 2006 Jan;31(1):178-81.	9
29 Barbe RP, Rubovszky G, Venturini-Andreoli A, Andreoli A. The treatment of borderline personality disorder patients with current suicidal behaviour. Clinical Neuropsychiatry: Journal of Treatment Evaluation. 2005 Sep;2(5):283-91.	6
30 Bartlett ML. The efficacy of no-suicide contracts with clients in counseling on an outpatient basis. Dissertation Abstracts International: Section B: The Sciences and Engineering. 2006;67(6-B):3438.	3
31 Basham C, Denneson LM, Millet L, Shen X, Duckart J, Dobscha SK. Characteristics and VA Health Care Utilization of U. S. Veterans Who Completed Suicide in Oregon Between 2000 and 2005. Suicide Life Threat Behav. 2011 Apr 4;42(3):287-96.	9

Excluded Trials	Exclusion Code
32 Bauer MS, Wisniewski SR, Kogan JN, Marangell LB, Thase ME, Sachs G. Brief report: paroxetine in younger and adult individuals at high risk for suicide. Psychopharmacol Bull. 2006;39(1):31-7.	3
33 Beasley CM, Jr., Ball SG, Nilsson ME, et al. Fluoxetine and adult suicidality revisited: an updated meta-analysis using expanded data sources from placebo-controlled trials. J Clin Psychopharmacol. 2007 Dec;27(6):682-6.	8
34 Beautrais A, Fergusson D, Coggan C, et al. Effective strategies for suicide prevention in New Zealand: a review of the evidence. N Z Med J. 2007;120(1251):U2459.	6
35 Beautrais AL, Fergusson DM, Horwood LJ. Firearms legislation and reductions in firearm-related suicide deaths in New Zealand. Aust N Z J Psychiatry. 2006 Mar;40(3):253-9.	4
36 Beautrais AL, Gibb SJ, Fergusson DM, Horwood LJ, Larkin GL. Removing bridge barriers stimulates suicides: an unfortunate natural experiment. Aust N Z J Psychiatry. 2009 Jun;43(6):495-7.	4
37 Bennewith O, Nowers M, Gunnell D. Effect of barriers on the Clifton suspension bridge, England, on local patterns of suicide: implications for prevention. Br J Psychiatry. 2007 Mar;190:266-7.	4
38 Berard R, Fong R, Carpenter DJ, Thomason C, Wilkinson C. An international, multicenter, placebo-controlled trial of paroxetine in adolescents with major depressive disorder. J Child Adolesc Psychopharmacol. 2006 Feb-Apr;16(1-2):59-75.	2
39 Bergen H, Hawton K, Murphy E, et al. Trends in prescribing and self-poisoning in relation to UK regulatory authority warnings against use of SSRI antidepressants in under-18-year-olds. Br J Clin Pharmacol. 2009 Oct;68(4):618-29.	9
40 Bergman J, Miodownik C, Palatnik A, Lerner V. Efficacy of bupropion XR in treatment-resistant elderly patients: a case series study. Clin Neuropharmacol. 2011 Jan-Feb;34(1):17-20.	9
41 Bergmans Y, Links PS. Reducing potential risk factors for suicide-related behavior with a group intervention for clients with recurrent suicide-related behavior. Ann Clin Psychiatry. 2009 Jan-Mar;21(1):17-25.	3
42 Bessant M, King EA, Peveler R. Characteristics of suicides in recent contact with NHS Direct. Psychiatric Bulletin. 2008 Mar;32(3):92-5.	9
43 Borschmann, Rohan, Henderson, et al. Crisis interventions for people with borderline personality disorder [Protocol]. Cochrane Database of Systematic Reviews. 2011 (10).	6
44 Bridge JA, Barbe RP, Birmaher B, Kolko DJ, Brent DA. Emergent suicidality in a clinical psychotherapy trial for adolescent depression. Am J Psychiatry. 2005 Nov;162(11):2173-5.	9
45 Bronisch T. Depression and Suicide: Antidepressive Therapies in the Acute and Chronic Treatment of Unipolar and Bipolar Affective Disorders - Are they Preventive According to Suicide? Krankenhauspsychiatrie. 2005 Sep;16(Suppl1):27-33.	1
46 Brown C, Wyman PA, Brinales JM, Gibbons RD. The role of randomized trials in testing interventions for the prevention of youth suicide. International Review of Psychiatry. 2007 Dec;19(6):617-31.	5
47 Burns J, Dudley M, Hazell P, Patton G. Clinical management of deliberate self-harm in young people: the need for evidence-based approaches to reduce repetition. Australian and New Zealand Journal of Psychiatry. 2005;39(3):121-8.	7
48 Cardish RJ. Psychopharmacologic management of suicidality in personality disorders. Can J Psychiatry. 2007 Jun;52(6 Suppl 1):115S-27S.	6
49 Carr A. Depression in young people: description, assessment and evidence-based treatment. Dev Neurorehabil. 2008 Jan-Mar;11(1):3-15.	6
50 Catanese AA, John MS, Di Battista J, Clarke DM. Acute cognitive therapy in reducing suicide risk following a presentation to an emergency department. Behaviour Change. 2009 May;26(1):16-26.	9

Excluded Trials	Exclusion Code
51 Chiesa M, Fonagy P, Gordon J. Community-based psychodynamic treatment program for severe personality disorders: clinical description and naturalistic evaluation. J Psychiatr Pract. 2009 Jan;15(1):12-24.	9
52 Chisholm D, van Ommeren M, Ayuso-Mateos JL, Saxena S. Cost-effectiveness of clinical interventions for reducing the global burden of bipolar disorder. Br J Psychiatry. 2005 Dec;187:559-67.	9
53 Cipriani A, Barbui C, Geddes JR. Suicide, depression, and antidepressants. BMJ. 2005;330(7488):373-4.	6
54 Cipriani A, Geddes JR, Furukawa TA, Barbui C. Metareview on short-term effectiveness and safety of antidepressants for depression: an evidence-based approach to inform clinical practice. Can J Psychiatry. 2007 Sep;52(9):553-62.	6
55 Cipriani A, Rendell JM, Geddes JR. Haloperidol alone or in combination for acute mania. Cochrane Database Syst Rev. 2006;3:CD004362.	3
56 Coffey CE. Building a system of perfect depression care in behavioral health. Jt Comm J Qual Patient Saf. 2007 Apr;33(4):193-9.	9
57 Cohen A, Houck PR, Szanto K, Dew MA, Gilman SE, Reynolds CF, III. Social inequalities in response to antidepressant treatment in older adults. Archives of General Psychiatry. 2006 Jan;63(1):50-6.	3
58 Cohen D. Should the use of selective serotonin reuptake inhibitors in child and adolescent depression be banned? Psychother Psychosom. 2007;76(1):5-14.	6
59 Cohen VK. Keeping students alive: mandating on-campus counseling saves suicidal college students' lives and limits liability. Fordham Law Rev. 2007 May;75(6):3081-135.	5
60 Combalbert N, Bourdet-Loubere S. Suicide by jumping and strategies to prevent it. L'Evolution Psychiatrique. 2006 Oct-Dec;71(4):685-95.	1
61 Combs H, Romm S. Psychiatric inpatient suicide: A literature review. Primary Psychiatry. 2007 Dec;14(12):67-74.	7
62 Comtois KA, Linehan MM. Psychosocial treatments of suicidal behaviors: a practice-friendly review. J Clin Psychol. 2006 Feb;62(2):161-70.	6
63 Cooper SL, Lezotte D, Jacobellis J, Diguiseppi C. Does availability of mental health resources prevent recurrent suicidal behavior? An ecological analysis. Suicide Life Threat Behav. 2006 Aug;36(4):409-17.	9
64 Corcoran J, Dattalo P, Crowley M, Brown E, Grindle L. A systematic review of psychosocial interventions for suicidal adolescents. Children and Youth Services Review. 2011 Nov;33(11):2112-8.	7
65 Coryell W. Maintenance treatment in bipolar disorder: A reassessment of lithium as the first choice. Bipolar Disorders. 2009 Jun;11(Suppl2):77-83.	6
66 Cottraux J, Note ID, Boutitie F, et al. Cognitive therapy versus Rogerian supportive therapy in borderline personality disorder. Two-year follow-up of a controlled pilot study. Psychother Psychosom. 2009;78(5):307-16.	2
67 Craig M, Howard L. Postnatal depression. Clin Evid (Online). 2009;2009.	7
68 Crawford MJ, Thomas O, Khan N, Kulinskaya E. Psychosocial interventions following self-harm: systematic review of their efficacy in preventing suicide. Br J Psychiatry. 2007 Jan;190:11-7.	7
69 Crits-Christoph P, Barber JP. Psychological treatments for personality disorders. Nathan, Peter E [Ed]. 2007:641-58.	6
70 Crocq MA, Naber D, Lader MH, et al. Suicide attempts in a prospective cohort of patients with schizophrenia treated with sertindole or risperidone. Eur Neuropsychopharmacol. 2010 Dec;20(12):829-38.	2

Excluded Trials	Exclusion Code
71 Currier GW, Fisher SG, Caine ED. Mobile crisis team intervention to enhance linkage of discharged suicidal emergency department patients to outpatient psychiatric services: a randomized controlled trial. Acad Emerg Med. 2010 Jan;17(1):36-43.	3
72 Cusimano MD, Sameem M. The effectiveness of middle and high school-based suicide prevention programmes for adolescents: a systematic review. Inj Prev. 2011 Feb;17(1):43-9.	4
73 Daigle MS, Daniel AE, Dear GE, et al. Preventing suicide in prisons, part II. International comparisons of suicide prevention services in correctional facilities. Crisis. 2007;28(3):122-30.	6
74 Daigle MS, Pouliot L, Chagnon F, Greenfield B, Mishara B. Suicide attempts: prevention of repetition. Can J Psychiatry. 2011 Oct;56(10):621-9.	7
75 Daigle MS. Suicide prevention through means restriction: Assessing the risk of substitution: A critical review and synthesis. Accident Analysis and Prevention. 2005 Jul;37(4):625-32.	6
76 Daniel SS, Goldston DB. Interventions for suicidal youth: A review of the literature and developmental considerations. Suicide and Life Threatening Behavior. 2009 Jun;39(3):252-68.	7
77 Daviss W. A review of co-morbid depression in pediatric ADHD: Etiologies, phenomenology, and treatment. Journal of Child and Adolescent Psychopharmacology. 2008 Dec;18(6):565-71.	6
78 De Leo D. The world health organization: Approach to evidence-based suicide prevention. Pompili, Maurizio [Ed]. 2011:55-64.	6
79 Denneson LM, Basham C, Dickinson KC, et al. Suicide risk assessment and content of VA health care contacts before suicide completion by veterans in Oregon. Psychiatr Serv. 2010 Dec;61(12):1192-7.	5
80 Department of Defense Task Force on the Prevention of Suicide by Members of the Armed Forces. The Challenge and the Promise: Strengthening the Force, Preventing Suicide and Saving Lives. Washington D.C.: Department of Defense; 2010.	6
81 Dixon L, Goldberg R, Iannone V, et al. Use of a critical time intervention to promote continuity of care after psychiatric inpatient hospitalization. Psychiatric Services. 2009;60(4):451-8.	3
82 Doering S, Horz S, Rentrop M, et al. Transference-focused psychotherapy v. treatment by community psychotherapists for borderline personality disorder: randomised controlled trial. Br J Psychiatry. 2010 May;196(5):389-95.	2
83 Doggrell SA. Fluoxetine--do the benefits outweigh the risks in adolescent major depression? Expert Opinion on Pharmacotherapy. 2005;6(1):147-50.	6
84 Dombrovski AY, Mulsant BH. The evidence for electroconvulsive therapy (ECT) in the treatment of severe late-life depression. ECT: the preferred treatment for severe depression in late life. Int Psychogeriatr. 2007 Feb;19(1):10-4, 27-35; discussion 24-6.	6
85 Dube P, Kurt K, Bair MJ, Theobald D, Williams LS. The p4 screener: evaluation of a brief measure for assessing potential suicide risk in 2 randomized effectiveness trials of primary care and oncology patients. Prim Care Companion J Clin Psychiatry. 2010;12(6).	9
86 Dubicka B, Hadley S, Roberts C. Suicidal behaviour in youths with depression treated with new-generation antidepressants: meta-analysis. Br J Psychiatry. 2006 Nov;189:393-8.	7
87 Dubicka B, Wilkinson P. Evidence-based treatment of adolescent major depression. Evid Based Ment Health. 2007 Nov;10(4):100-2.	6
88 Dudley M, Goldney R, Hadzi-Pavlovic D. Are adolescents dying by suicide taking SSRI antidepressants? A review of observational studies. Australasian Psychiatry. 2010 Jun;18(3):242-5.	7
89 Dudley M, Hadzi-Pavlovic D, Andrews D, Perich T. New-generation antidepressants, suicide and depressed adolescents: How should clinicians respond to changing evidence? Australian and New Zealand Journal of Psychiatry. 2008 Jun;42(6):456-66.	6

Excluded Trials	Exclusion Code
90 Ebmeier KP. No apparent difference in suicide risk between older and newer antidepressants although older drugs may increase risk of suicide attempt during the first month of treatment. Evid Based Ment Health. 2006 Aug;9(3):82.	5
91 Emslie GJ, Yeung PP, Kunz NR. Long-term, open-label venlafaxine extended-release treatment in children and adolescents with major depressive disorder. CNS Spectr. 2007 Mar;12(3):223-33.	9
92 Eskin M, Ertekin K, Demir H. Efficacy of a problem-solving therapy for depression and suicide potential in adolescents and young adults. Cognitive Therapy and Research. 2008 Apr;32(2):227-45.	2
93 Esposito-Smythers C, Spirito A, Uth R, LaChance H. Cognitive behavioral treatment for suicidal alcohol abusing adolescents: development and pilot testing. Am J Addict. 2006;15 Suppl 1:126-30.	9
94 Everly GS, Jr., Flynn BW. Principles and practical procedures for acute psychological first aid training for personnel without mental health experience. Int J Emerg Ment Health. 2006 Spring;8(2):93-100.	6
95 Fergusson D, Doucette S, Glass KC, et al. Association between suicide attempts and selective serotonin reuptake inhibitors: Systematic review of randomised controlled trials. BMJ: British Medical Journal. 2005 Feb;330(7488):396.	7
96 Fleischhaker C, Bohme R, Sixt B, Bruck C, Schneider C, Schulz E. Dialectical Behavioral Therapy for Adolescents (DBT-A): a clinical Trial for Patients with suicidal and self-injurious Behavior and Borderline Symptoms with a one-year Follow-up. Child Adolesc Psychiatry Ment Health. 2011;5(1):3.	9
97 Fleischmann A, Bertolote JM, Wasserman D, et al. Effectiveness of brief intervention and contact for suicide attempters: a randomized controlled trial in five countries. Bull World Health Organ. 2008 Sep;86(9):703-9.	2
98 Florentine JB, Crane C. Suicide prevention by limiting access to methods: A review of theory and practice. Social Science & Medicine. 2010 May;70(10):1626-32.	6
99 Fountoulakis KN, Gonda X, Siamouli M, Rihmer Z. Psychotherapeutic intervention and suicide risk reduction in bipolar disorder: a review of the evidence. J Affect Disord. 2009 Feb;113(1-2):21-9.	7
100 Fountoulakis KN, Grunze H, Panagiotidis P, Kaprinis G. Treatment of bipolar depression: An update. Journal of Affective Disorders. 2008 Jul;109(1-2):21-34.	6
101 Fountoulakis KN, Vieta E, Schmidt F. Aripiprazole monotherapy in the treatment of bipolar disorder: A meta-analysis. J Affect Disord. 2010 Oct 30.	7
102 Freeman SA. Suicide risk and psychopharmacology: assessment and management of acute and chronic risk factors. J Clin Psychiatry. 2009 Jul;70(7):1052-3.	6
103 Fu Y-X, Shen J-L, Dang W. Effects of psychological intervention on the young people of attempted suicide. Chinese Mental Health Journal. 2007 Aug;21(8):571-4.	1
104 Gardner W, Klima J, Chisolm D, et al. Screening, triage, and referral of patients who report suicidal thought during a primary care visit. Pediatrics. 2010 May;125(5):945-52.	3
105 Garvey KA, Penn JV, Campbell AL, Esposito-Smythers C, Spirito A. Contracting for safety with patients: Clinical practice and forensic implications. Journal of the American Academy of Psychiatry and the Law. 2009 Sep;37(3):363-70.	6
106 Geddes JR, Barbui C, Cipriani A. Risk of suicidal behaviour in adults taking antidepressants. BMJ. 2009;339:b3066.	5
107 Gilbert JW, Wheeler GR, Storey BB, et al. Suicidality in chronic noncancer pain patients. Int J Neurosci. 2009;119(10):1968-79.	9

Excluded Trials	Exclusion Code
108 Glass JE, Ilgen MA, Winters JJ, Murray RL, Perron BE, Chermack ST. Inpatient hospitalization in addiction treatment for patients with a history of suicide attempt: A case of support for treatment performance measures. Journal of Psychoactive Drugs. 2010 Sep;42(3):315-25.	3
109 Goldney RD. Suicide Prevention: A Pragmatic Review of Recent Studies. Crisis: The Journal of Crisis Intervention and Suicide Prevention. 2005;26(3):128-40.	6
110 Goldstein BI, Bukstein OG. Comorbid substance use disorders among youth with bipolar disorder: opportunities for early identification and prevention. J Clin Psychiatry. 2010 Mar;71(3):348-58.	6
111 Gottman JM, Gottman JS, Atkins CL. The Comprehensive Soldier Fitness Program: Family skills component. American Psychologist. 2011 Jan;66(1):52-7.	6
112 Gould MS, Kalafat J, Harrismunfakh JL, Kleinman M. An evaluation of crisis hotline outcomes. Part 2: Suicidal callers. Suicide Life Threat Behav. 2007 Jun;37(3):338-52.	9
113 Grandjean EM, Aubry JM. Lithium: updated human knowledge using an evidence-based approach: Part I: Clinical efficacy in bipolar disorder. CNS Drugs. 2009;23(3):225-40.	7
114 Grawe R, Falloon I, Widen J, Skogvoll E. Two years of continued early treatment for recent-onset schizophrenia: A randomised controlled study. Acta Psychiatrica Scandinavica. 2006 Nov;114(5):328-36.	2
115 Greden JF, Valenstein M, Spinner J, et al. Buddy-to-Buddy, a citizen soldier peer support program to counteract stigma, PTSD, depression, and suicide. Ann N Y Acad Sci. 2010 Oct;1208:90-7.	4
116 Gutierrez PM, Brenner LA, Olson-Madden JH, et al. Consultation as a means of veteran suicide prevention. Professional Psychology: Research and Practice. 2009 Dec;40(6):586-92.	6
117 Guzzetta F, Tondo L, Centorrino F, Baldessarini RJ. Lithium treatment reduces suicide risk in recurrent major depressive disorder. J Clin Psychiatry. 2007 Mar;68(3):380-3.	7
118 Gyorgy P, Zoltan R. The role of sleep-improving and anxiolytic effect of mirtazapine in decreasing suicide risk in patients with depression. Psychiatria Hungarica. 2009;24(Suppl):6-11.	1
119 Haffner WH. Veteran suicide. Mil Med. 2010 Oct;175(10):i.	6
120 Hall WD, Lucke J. How have the selective serotonin reuptake inhibitor antidepressants affected suicide mortality? Australian and New Zealand Journal of Psychiatry. 2006 Nov;40(11-12):941-50.	7
121 Hamilton SM, Rolf KA. Suicide in adolescent American Indians: Preventative social work programs. Child & Adolescent Social Work Journal. 2010 Aug;27(4):283-90.	6
122 Hammad TA, Laughren T, Racoosin J. Suicidality in pediatric patients treated with antidepressant drugs. Arch Gen Psychiatry. 2006 Mar;63(3):332-9.	3
123 Hammad TA, Laughren TP, Racoosin JA. Suicide rates in short-term randomized controlled trials of newer antidepressants. J Clin Psychopharmacol. 2006 Apr;26(2):203-7.	8
124 Hammerness PG, Vivas FM, Geller DA. Selective serotonin reuptake inhibitors in pediatric psychopharmacology: a review of the evidence. J Pediatr. 2006 Feb;148(2):158-65.	7
125 Hampton T. Depression care effort brings dramatic drop in large HMO population's suicide rate. JAMA: Journal of the American Medical Association. 2010 May;303(19):1903-5.	6
126 Hamrin V, Scahill L. Selective serotonin reuptake inhibitors for children and adolescents with major depression: current controversies and recommendations. Issues Ment Health Nurs. 2005 May;26(4):433-50.	6
127 Han D, Wang EC. Remission from depression: A review of venlafaxine clinical and economic evidence. Pharmacoeconomics. 2005;23(6):567-81.	6

Excluded Trials	Exclusion Code
128 Harned MS, Chapman AL, Dexter-Mazza ET, Murray A, Comtois KA, Linehan MM. Treating co-occurring Axis I disorders in recurrently suicidal women with borderline personality disorder: a 2-year randomized trial of dialectical behavior therapy versus community treatment by experts. J Consult Clin Psychol. 2008 Dec;76(6):1068-75.	3
129 Harrison-Woolrych M. Varenicline and suicide. Safety data from New Zealand. BMJ. 2009;339:b5654.	6
130 Harrod, Curtis S, Goss, et al. Interventions for primary prevention of suicide in the post-secondary educational setting [Protocol]. Cochrane Database of Systematic Reviews. 2011 (11).	6
131 Harter M, Bermejo I, Ollenschlager G, et al. Improving quality of care for depression: the German Action Programme for the implementation of evidence-based guidelines. Int J Qual Health Care. 2006 Apr;18(2):113-9.	2
132 Hassanian-Moghaddam H, Sarjami S, Kolahi AA, Carter GL. Postcards in Persia: randomised controlled trial to reduce suicidal behaviours 12 months after hospital-treated self-poisoning. Br J Psychiatry. 2011 Feb 22;198:309-16.	2
133 Haukka J, Arffman M, Partonen T, et al. Antidepressant use and mortality in Finland: a register-linkage study from a nationwide cohort. Eur J Clin Pharmacol. 2009 Jul;65(7):715-20.	2
134 Haukka J, Tiihonen J, Harkanen T, Lonnqvist J. Association between medication and risk of suicide, attempted suicide and death in nationwide cohort of suicidal patients with schizophrenia. Pharmacoepidemiol Drug Saf. 2008 Jul;17(7):686-96.	2
135 Hawgood J, De Leo D. Anxiety disorders and suicidal behaviour: an update. Curr Opin Psychiatry. 2008 Jan;21(1):51-64.	7
136 Hays JT, Ebbert JO. Adverse effects and tolerability of medications for the treatment of tobacco use and dependence. Drugs. 2010 Dec 24;70(18):2357-72.	6
137 Hazell P. Depression in children and adolescents. Clin Evid (Online). 2009;2009.	3
138 Hazell P. Depression in children and adolescents. Clin Evid (Online). 2011;2011.	7
139 Heisel MJ, Duberstein PR. Suicide Prevention in Older Adults. Clinical Psychology: Science and Practice. 2005 Fal;12(3):242-59.	6
140 Hennen J, Baldessarini RJ. Suicidal risk during treatment with clozapine: A meta-analysis. Schizophrenia Research. 2005 Mar;73(2-3):139-45.	6
141 Hesdorffer DC, Berg AT, Kanner AM. An update on antiepileptic drugs and suicide: are there definitive answers yet? Epilepsy Curr. 2010 Nov;10(6):137-45.	6
142 Hong J, Reed C, Novick D, Haro JM, Aguado J. Clinical and economic consequences of medication non-adherence in the treatment of patients with a manic/mixed episode of bipolar disorder: Results from the European Mania in Bipolar Longitudinal Evaluation of Medication (EMBLEM) Study. Psychiatry Res. 2011 May 14.	2
143 Hough D, Lewis P. A suicide prevention advisory group at an academic medical center. Mil Med. 2010 May;175(5):347-51.	6
144 Hughes S, Cohen D. A systematic review of long-term studies of drug treated and non-drug treated depression. Journal of Affective Disorders. 2009;118(1-3):9-18.	3
145 Hur JW, Kim WJ, Kim YK. The Mediating Effect of Psychosocial Factors on Suicidal Probability among Adolescents. Arch Suicide Res. 2011 Oct;15(4):327-36.	1
146 Ilgen MA, Jain A, Lucas E, Moos RH. Substance use-disorder treatment and a decline in attempted suicide during and after treatment. J Stud Alcohol Drugs. 2007 Jul;68(4):503-9.	9
147 Ille R, Spona J, Zickl M, et al. "Add-On"-therapy with an individualized preparation consisting of free amino acids for patients with a major depression. European Archives of Psychiatry and Clinical Neuroscience. 2007 Jun;257(4):222-9.	2

Excluded Trials	Exclusion Code
148 Innamorati M, Pompili M, Amore M, et al. Suicide prevention in late life: Is there sound evidence for practice? In: Pompili M, Tatarelli R, eds. Evidence-based practice in suicidology: A source book. Cambridge, MA: Hogrefe Publishing; 2011:211-32.	7
149 Irons J. Fluvoxamine in the treatment of anxiety disorders. Neuropsychiatr Dis Treat. 2005 Dec;1(4):289-99.	6
150 Isaac M, Elias B, Katz LY, et al. Gatekeeper training as a preventative intervention for suicide: a systematic review. Can J Psychiatry. 2009 Apr;54(4):260-8.	4
151 Jacono J, Jacono B. The use of puppetry for health promotion and suicide prevention among Mi'Kmaq youth. J Holist Nurs. 2008 Mar;26(1):50-5.	6
152 Jakupcak M, Varra EM. Treating Iraq and Afghanistan war veterans with PTSD who are at high risk for suicide. Cognitive and Behavioral Practice. 2011 Feb;18(1):85-97.	6
153 Jones G, Gavrilovic JJ, McCabe R, Becktas C, Priebe S. Treating suicidal patients in an acute psychiatric day hospital: a challenge to assumptions about risk and overnight care. Journal of Mental Health. 2008;17(4):375-87.	3
154 Jorm AF, Kelly CM, Morgan AJ. Participant distress in psychiatric research: a systematic review. Psychol Med. 2007 Jul;37(7):917-26.	3
155 Juurlink DN, Mamdani MM, Kopp A, Redelmeier DA. The risk of suicide with selective serotonin reuptake inhibitors in the elderly. Am J Psychiatry. 2006 May;163(5):813-21.	9
156 Kaizar EE, Greenhouse JB, Seltman H, Kelleher K. Do antidepressants cause suicidality in children? A Bayesian meta-analysis. Clin Trials. 2006;3(2):73-90; discussion 1-8.	8
157 Kanner AM. Depression and epilepsy: A review of multiple facets of their close relation. Neurologic Clinics. 2009 Nov;27(4):865-80.	6
158 Karayal ON, Anway SD, Batzar E, Vanderburg DG. Assessments of suicidality in double-blind, placebo-controlled trials of ziprasidone. J Clin Psychiatry. 2011 Mar;72(3):367-75.	6
159 Kaslow NJ, Leiner AS, Reviere S, et al. Suicidal, abused African American women's response to a culturally informed intervention. Journal of Consulting and Clinical Psychology. 2010 Aug;78(4):449-58.	3
160 Kasper S, Montgomery SA, Moller HJ, et al. Longitudinal analysis of the suicidal behaviour risk in short-term placebo-controlled studies of mirtazapine in major depressive disorder. World J Biol Psychiatry. 2010 Feb;11(1):36-44.	3
161 Kennard BD, Silva SG, Mayes TL, et al. Assessment of safety and long-term outcomes of initial treatment with placebo in TADS. The American Journal of Psychiatry. 2009 Mar;166(3):337-44.	3
162 Kennedy CH, Cook JH, Poole DR, Brunson CL, Jones DE. Review of the first year of an overseas military gambling treatment program. Mil Med. 2005 Aug;170(8):683-7.	9
163 Kennedy SH, Giacobbe P, Rizvi SJ, et al. Deep brain stimulation for treatment-resistant depression: follow-up after 3 to 6 years. Am J Psychiatry. 2011 May;168(5):502-10.	9
164 Keshtkar M, Ghanizadeh A, Firoozabadi A. Repetitive Transcranial Magnetic Stimulation Versus Electroconvulsive Therapy for the Treatment of Major Depressive Disorder, A Randomized Controlled Clinical Trial. J ECT. 2011 Nov 9.	2
165 Kessing LV, Sondergard L, Kvist K, Andersen PK. Suicide risk in patients treated with lithium. Arch Gen Psychiatry. 2005 Aug;62(8):860-6.	2
166 Kim HM, Eisenberg D, Ganoczy D, et al. Examining the relationship between clinical monitoring and suicide risk among patients with depression: matched case-control study and instrumental variable approaches. Health Serv Res. 2010 Oct;45(5 Pt 1):1205-26.	9
167 Klein DF. The flawed basis for FDA post-marketing safety decisions: the example of anti-depressants and children. Neuropsychopharmacology. 2006 Apr;31(4):689-99.	6
168 Knox KL, Pflanz S, Talcott GW, et al. The US Air Force suicide prevention program: implications for public health policy. Am J Public Health. 2010 Dec;100(12):2457-63.	9

Excluded Trials	Exclusion Code
169 Koehn CV, Cutcliffe JR. Hope and interpersonal psychiatric/mental health nursing: a systematic review of the literature--part one. J Psychiatr Ment Health Nurs. 2007 Apr;14(2):134-40.	7
170 Kolla NJ, Eisenberg H, Links PS. Epidemiology, risk factors, and psychopharmacological management of suicidal behavior in borderline personality disorder. Archives of Suicide Research. 2008 Jan;12(1):1-19.	7
171 Konrad N, Daigle MS, Daniel AE, et al. Preventing suicide in prisons, part I. Recommendations from the International Association for Suicide Prevention Task Force on Suicide in Prisons. Crisis. 2007;28(3):113-21.	6
172 Kostenuik M, Ratnapalan M. Approach to adolescent suicide prevention. Can Fam Physician. 2010 Aug;56(8):755-60.	6
173 Kratochvil CJ, Vitiello B, Walkup J, et al. Selective serotonin reuptake inhibitors in pediatric depression: is the balance between benefits and risks favorable? J Child Adolesc Psychopharmacol. 2006 Feb-Apr;16(1-2):11-24.	8
174 Kryzhanovskaya LA, Robertson-Plouch CK, Xu W, Carlson JL, Merida KM, Dittmann RW. The safety of olanzapine in adolescents with schizophrenia or bipolar I disorder: a pooled analysis of 4 clinical trials. J Clin Psychiatry. 2009 Feb;70(2):247-58.	6
175 Kutcher S, Gardner DM. Use of selective serotonin reuptake inhibitors and youth suicide: Making sense from a confusing story. Current Opinion in Psychiatry. 2008 Jan;21(1):65-9.	6
176 Lapierre S, Dube M, Bouffard L, Alain M. Addressing suicidal ideations through the realization of meaningful personal goals. Crisis. 2007;28(1):16-25.	3
177 Lapierre S, Erlangsen A, Waern M, et al. A systematic review of elderly suicide prevention programs. Crisis. 2011 Jan 1;32(2):88-98.	7
178 Lauterbach E, Felber W, Muller-Oerlinghausen B, et al. Adjunctive lithium treatment in the prevention of suicidal behaviour in depressive disorders: a randomised, placebo-controlled, 1-year trial. Acta Psychiatr Scand. 2008 Dec;118(6):469-79.	2
179 Leenaars AA. Evidence-based psychotherapy with suicidal people: A systematic review. Pompili, Maurizio [Ed]. 2011:89-123.	7
180 Leenaars AA. Psychotherapy with Suicidal People: The Commonalities. Archives of Suicide Research. 2006 Dec;10(4):305-22.	6
181 Leon AC, Solomon DA, Li C, et al. Antidepressants and risks of suicide and suicide attempts: a 27-year observational study. Journal of Clinical Psychiatry. 2011;72(5):580-6.	9
182 Lester D. Resources and Tactics for Preventing Suicide. Clinical Neuropsychiatry: Journal of Treatment Evaluation. 2005 Feb;2(1):32-6.	5
183 Lester D. The use of the Internet for counseling the suicidal individual: possibilities and drawbacks. Omega (Westport). 2008;58(3):233-50.	6
184 Levy KN, Meehan KB, Yeomans FE. Transference-focused psychotherapy reduces treatment drop-out and suicide attempters compared with community psychotherapist treatment in borderline personality disorder. Evid Based Ment Health. 2010 Nov;13(4):119.	2
185 Lewis LM. No-harm contracts: A review of what we know. Suicide and Life Threatening Behavior. 2007 Feb;37(1):50-7.	6
186 Licinio J, Wong M-L. Depression, antidepressants and suicidality: a critical appraisal. Nat Rev Drug Discov. 2005;4(2):165-71.	6
187 Links PS, Hoffman B. Preventing suicidal behaviour in a general hospital psychiatric service: priorities for programming. Can J Psychiatry. 2005 Jul;50(8):490-6.	7
188 Lizardi D, Stanley B. Treatment engagement: A neglected aspect in the psychiatric care of suicidal patients. Psychiatric Services. 2010 Dec;61(12):1183-91.	7
189 Long CG, Fulton B, Dolley O, Hollin CR. Dealing with Feelings: the effectiveness of cognitive behavioural group treatment for women in secure settings. Behav Cogn Psychother. 2011 Mar;39(2):243-7.	9

Excluded Trials	Exclusion Code
190 Lorillard S, Schmitt L, Andreoli A. How to treat deliberate self-harm: From clinical research to effective treatment choice? Part 1: An update treatment efficacy among unselected patients referred to emergency room with deliberate self-harm. Annales Medico-Psychologiques. 2011 May;169(4):221-8.	1
191 Lorillard S, Schmitt L, Andreoli A. How to treat suicide attempt? Part 2: A review of treatments and their efficiency among borderline personality disorder patients. Annales Medico-Psychologiques. 2011 May;169(4):229-36.	1
192 Lu YJ, Chang HJ, Tung YY, Hsu MC, Lin MF. Alleviating psychological distress of suicide survivors: evaluation of a volunteer care programme. J Psychiatr Ment Health Nurs. 2011 Jun;18(5):449-56.	3
193 Ludwig J, Marcotte DE, Norberg K. Anti-depressants and suicide. J Health Econ. 2009 May;28(3):659-76.	2
194 Lynch MA, Howard PB, El-Mallakh P, Matthews JM. Assessment and management of hospitalized suicidal patients. J Psychosoc Nurs Ment Health Serv. 2008 Jul;46(7):45-52.	6
195 Malmberg, Lena, Fenton, Mark, Rathbone, John. Individual psychodynamic psychotherapy and psychoanalysis for schizophrenia and severe mental illness [Systematic Review]. Cochrane Database of Systematic Reviews. 2010 (3).	3
196 Malone D, Newron-Howes G, Simmonds S, Marriot S, Tyrer P. Community mental health teams (CMHTs) for people with severe mental illnesses and disordered personality. Cochrane Database Syst Rev. 2007 (3):CD000270.	3
197 Mamo DC. Managing suicidality in schizophrenia. Can J Psychiatry. 2007 Jun;52(6 Suppl 1):59S-70S.	7
198 Mann J, Currier D. Evidence-based suicide prevention strategies: An overview. Pompili, Maurizio [Ed]. 2011:67-87.	6
199 Manna M. Effectiveness of formal observation in inpatient psychiatry in preventing adverse outcomes: The state of the science. Journal of Psychiatric and Mental Health Nursing. 2010 Apr;17(3):268-73.	7
200 Manthorpe J, Iliffe S. Social work with older people--Reducing suicide risk: A critical review of practice and prevention. British Journal of Social Work. 2011 Jan;41(1):131-47.	6
201 Marangell LB, Dennehy EB, Wisniewski SR, et al. Case-control analyses of the impact of pharmacotherapy on prospectively observed suicide attempts and completed suicides in bipolar disorder: findings from STEP-BD. J Clin Psychiatry. 2008 Jun;69(6):916-22.	9
202 March JS, Klee BJ, Kremer CM. Treatment benefit and the risk of suicidality in multicenter, randomized, controlled trials of sertraline in children and adolescents. J Child Adolesc Psychopharmacol. 2006 Feb-Apr;16(1-2):91-102.	8
203 Matakas F, Rohrbach E. Suicide prevention in the psychiatric hospital. Suicide Life Threat Behav. 2007 Oct;37(5):507-17.	2
204 McAuliffe N, Perry L. Making it safer: a health centre's strategy for suicide prevention. Psychiatr Q. 2007 Dec;78(4):295-307.	3
205 McElroy SL, Kotwal R, Kaneria R, Keck PE, Jr. Antidepressants and suicidal behavior in bipolar disorder. Bipolar Disorders. 2006 Oct;8(5 pt 2):596-617.	7
206 McMain S. Effectiveness of psychosocial treatments on suicidality in personality disorders. Can J Psychiatry. 2007 Jun;52(6 Suppl 1):103S-14S.	7
207 McQuillan A, Nicastro R, Guenot F, Girard M, Lissner C, Ferrero F. Intensive Dialectical Behavior Therapy for Outpatients With Borderline Personality Disorder Who Are in Crisis. Psychiatric Services. 2005 Feb;56(2):193-7.	2
208 Melle I, Johannessen JO, Friis S, et al. Course and predictors of suicidality over the first two years of treatment in first-episode schizophrenia spectrum psychosis. Arch Suicide Res. 2010 Apr;14(2):158-70.	2

Excluded Trials	Exclusion Code
209 Melvin GA, Tonge BJ, King NJ, Heyne D, Gordon MS, Klimkeit E. A comparison of cognitive-behavioral therapy, sertraline, and their combination for adolescent depression. Journal of the American Academy of Child & Adolescent Psychiatry. 2006;45(10):1151-61.	3
210 Merrick J, Merrick E, Lunsky Y, Kandel I. Review of suicidality in persons with intellectual disability. Israel Journal of Psychiatry and Related Sciences. 2006;43(4):258-64.	6
211 Mishara BL, Chagnon F, Daigle M, et al. Which helper behaviors and intervention styles are related to better short-term outcomes in telephone crisis intervention? Results from a Silent Monitoring Study of Calls to the U.S. 1-800-SUICIDE Network. Suicide Life Threat Behav. 2007 Jun;37(3):308-21.	3
212 Mishara BL, Houle J, Lavoie B. Comparison of the effects of four suicide prevention programs for family and friends of high-risk suicidal men who do not seek help themselves. Suicide Life Threat Behav. 2005 Jun;35(3):329-42.	9
213 Mitchell SA. Examining the effectiveness of a school-based mental health center's services. Dissertation Abstracts International Section A: Humanities and Social Sciences. 2008;68(8-A):3282.	3
214 Moller HJ. Evidence for beneficial effects of antidepressants on suicidality in depressive patients: a systematic review. Eur Arch Psychiatry Clin Neurosci. 2006 Sep;256(6):329-43.	6
215 Morriss R, Gask L, Webb R, Dixon C, Appleby L. The effects on suicide rates of an educational intervention for front-line health professionals with suicidal patients (the STORM Project). Psychol Med. 2005 Jul;35(7):957-60.	4
216 Mortimer AM, Singh P, Shepherd CJ, Puthiryackal J. Clozapine for treatment-resistant schizophrenia: National Institute of Clinical Excellence (NICE) guidance in the real world. Clin Schizophr Relat Psychoses. 2010 Apr;4(1):49-55.	3
217 Mosholder AD, Willy M. Suicidal adverse events in pediatric randomized, controlled clinical trials of antidepressant drugs are associated with active drug treatment: a meta-analysis. J Child Adolesc Psychopharmacol. 2006 Feb-Apr;16(1-2):25-32.	8
218 Mowla A, Kardeh E. Topiramate augmentation in patients with resistant major depressive disorder: a double-blind placebo-controlled clinical trial. Prog Neuropsychopharmacol Biol Psychiatry. 2011 Jun 1;35(4):970-3.	2
219 Mulder RT, Joyce PR, Frampton CM, Luty SE. Antidepressant treatment is associated with a reduction in suicidal ideation and suicide attempts. Acta Psychiatr Scand. 2008 Aug;118(2):116-22.	9
220 Muller-Oerlinghausen B, Felber W, Berghofer A, Lauterbach E, Ahrens B. The Impact of Lithium Long-Term Medication on Suicidal Behavior and Mortality of Bipolar Patients. Archives of Suicide Research. 2005 Sep;9(3):307-19.	6
221 Muller-Oerlinghausen B, Lewitzka U. Lithium reduces pathological aggression and suicidality: A mini-review. Neuropsychobiology. 2010 Jun;62(1):43-9.	6
222 Musselman DL, Somerset WI, Guo Y, et al. A double-blind, multicenter, parallel-group study of paroxetine, desipramine, or placebo in breast cancer patients (stages I, II, III, and IV) with major depression. Journal of Clinical Psychiatry. 2006;67(2):288-96.	3
223 Najavits LM, Schmitz M, Gotthardt S, Weiss RD. Seeking safety plus exposure therapy: An outcome study on dual diagnosis men. Journal of Psychoactive Drugs. 2005 Dec;37(4):425-35.	9
224 Nakagawa M, Yamada T, Yamada S, Natori M, Hirayasu Y, Kawanishi C. Follow-up study of suicide attempters who were given crisis intervention during hospital stay: Pilot study. Psychiatry and Clinical Neurosciences. 2009 Feb;63(1):122-3.	6
225 Navarro-Mancilla AA, Rueda-Jaimes GE. Internet Addiction: A Critical Review of the Literature. Revista Colombiana de Psiquiatria. 2007 Dec;36(4):691-700.	1
226 Naylor PB, Cowie HA, Walters SJ, Talamelli L, Dawkins J. Impact of a mental health teaching programme on adolescents. Br J Psychiatry. 2009 Apr;194(4):365-70.	3

Excluded Trials	Exclusion Code
227 Neacsiu AD, Rizvi SL, Linehan MM. Dialectical behavior therapy skills use as a mediator and outcome of treatment for borderline personality disorder. Behaviour Research and Therapy. 2010 Sep;48(9):832-9.	9
228 Nelson JC, Delucchi K, Schneider L. Suicidal thinking and behavior during treatment with sertraline in late-life depression. Am J Geriatr Psychiatry. 2007 Jul;15(7):573-80.	3
229 Olmsted CL, Kockler DR. Topiramate for alcohol dependence. Ann Pharmacother. 2008 Oct;42(10):1475-80.	7
230 Omar HA. A model program for youth suicide prevention. Int J Adolesc Med Health. 2005 Jul-Sep;17(3):275-8.	4
231 Oordt MS, Jobes DA, Rudd M, et al. Development of a Clinical Guide to Enhance Care for Suicidal Patients. Professional Psychology: Research and Practice. 2005 Apr;36(2):208-18.	6
232 Oquendo MA, Chaudhury SR, Mann J. Pharmacotherapy of Suicidal Behavior in Bipolar Disorder. Archives of Suicide Research. 2005 Sep;9(3):237-50.	6
233 Owens C, Lambert H, Donovan J, Lloyd KR. A qualitative study of help seeking and primary care consultation prior to suicide. Br J Gen Pract. 2005 Jul;55(516):503-9.	3
234 Owens C, Owen G, Lambert H, et al. Public involvement in suicide prevention: understanding and strengthening lay responses to distress. BMC Public Health. 2009;9:308.	3
235 Oxman TE, Dietrich AJ, Schulberg HC. Evidence-based models of integrated management of depression in primary care. Psychiatr Clin North Am. 2005 Dec;28(4):1061-77.	6
236 Page SA, King MC. No-suicide agreements: current practices and opinions in a Canadian urban health region. Can J Psychiatry. 2008 Mar;53(3):169-76.	3
237 Palmer S. Suicide statistics for the UK and the National Suicide Prevention Strategy. Palmer, Stephen [Ed]. 2008:27-47.	6
238 Parellada M, Saiz P, Moreno D, et al. Is attempted suicide different in adolescent and adults? Psychiatry Res. 2008 Jan 15;157(1-3):131-7.	2
239 Pasieczny N, Connor J. The effectiveness of dialectical behaviour therapy in routine public mental health settings: An Australian controlled trial. Behaviour Research and Therapy. 2011 Jan;49(1):4-10.	9
240 Pena JB, Caine ED. Screening as an Approach for Adolescent Suicide Prevention. Suicide and Life Threatening Behavior. 2006 Dec;36(6):614-37.	7
241 Perahia DGS, Wang F, Mallinckrodt CH, Walker DJ, Detke MJ. Duloxetine in the treatment of major depressive disorder: a placebo- and paroxetine-controlled trial. European Psychiatry: the Journal of the Association of European Psychiatrists. 2006;21(6):367-78.	2
242 Phelan JC, Sinkewicz M, Castille DM, Huz S, Muenzenmaier K, Link BG. Effectiveness and outcomes of assisted outpatient treatment in New York State. Psychiatr Serv. 2010 Feb;61(2):137-43.	3
243 Phillips KA. Suicidality in body dysmorphic disorder. Primary Psychiatry. 2007 Dec;14(12):58-66.	6
244 Pirruccello LM. Preventing adolescent suicide: a community takes action. J Psychosoc Nurs Ment Health Serv. 2010 May;48(5):34-41.	6
245 Pompili M, Innamorati M, Girardi P, Tatarelli R, Lester D. Evidence-based interventions for preventing suicide in youths. In: Pompili M, Tatarelli R, eds. Evidence-based practice in suicidology: A source book. Cambridge, MA: Hogrefe Publishing; 2011:171-209.	7
246 Pompili M, Innamorati M, Tatarelli R. Suicide and anorexia nervosa. Minerva Psichiatrica. 2007 Dec;48(4):387-96.	1
247 Poon LH, Kang GA, Lee AJ. Role of tetrabenazine for Huntington's disease-associated chorea. Ann Pharmacother. 2010 Jun;44(6):1080-9.	5
248 Portzky G, van Heeringen K. Suicide prevention in adolescents: a controlled study of the effectiveness of a school-based psycho-educational program. J Child Psychol Psychiatry. 2006 Sep;47(9):910-8.	2

Excluded Trials	Exclusion Code
249 Posner K, Oquendo MA, Gould M, Stanley B, Davies M. Columbia Classification Algorithm of Suicide Assessment (C-CASA): classification of suicidal events in the FDA's pediatric suicidal risk analysis of antidepressants. Am J Psychiatry. 2007 Jul;164(7):1035-43.	6
250 Posternak MA, Zimmerman M. Therapeutic effect of follow-up assessments on antidepressant and placebo response rates in antidepressant efficacy trials: meta-analysis. British Journal of Psychiatry. 2007;190:287-92.	7
251 Power L, Morgan S, Byrne S, et al. A pilot study evaluating a support programme for parents of young people with suicidal behaviour. Child and Adolescent Psychiatry and Mental Health. 2009 Jul;3:20.	3
252 Prabhu SL, Molinari V, Bowers T, Lomax J. Role of the family in suicide prevention: An attachment and family systems perspective. Bulletin of the Menninger Clinic. 2010 Fal;74(4):301-27.	7
253 Prendergast N, McCausland J. Dialectic behaviour therapy: A 12-month collaborative program in a local community setting. Behaviour Change. 2007 Mar;24(1):25-35.	9
254 Raja M, Azzoni A, Koukopoulos AE. Psychopharmacological treatment before suicide attempt among patients admitted to a psychiatric intensive care unit. J Affect Disord. 2009 Feb;113(1-2):37-44.	2
255 Raja M, Azzoni A. Are antidepressants warranted in the treatment of patients who present suicidal behavior? Hum Psychopharmacol. 2008 Dec;23(8):661-8.	2
256 Read J, Bentall R. The effectiveness of electroconvulsive therapy: a literature review. Epidemiol Psichiatr Soc. 2010 Oct-Dec;19(4):333-47.	7
257 Reardon CL, Factor RM. Sport psychiatry: a systematic review of diagnosis and medical treatment of mental illness in athletes. Sports Med. 2010 Nov 1;40(11):961-80.	6
258 Redden L, Pritchett Y, Robieson W, et al. Suicidality and divalproex sodium: Analysis of controlled studies in multiple indications. Annals of General Psychiatry. 2011 Jan;10:1.	8
259 Reeves H, Batra S, May RS, Zhang R, Dahl DC, Li X. Efficacy of risperidone augmentation to antidepressants in the management of suicidality in major depressive disorder: a randomized, double-blind, placebo-controlled pilot study. J Clin Psychiatry. 2008 Aug;69(8):1228-336.	3
260 Reeves RR, Ladner ME. Antidepressant-induced suicidality: An update. CNS Neuroscience & Therapeutics. 2010 Aug;16(4):227-34.	6
261 Reyes VA, Hicklin TA. Anger in the combat zone. Mil Med. 2005 Jun;170(6):483-7.	6
262 Rhee WK, Merbaum M, Strube MJ, Self SM. Efficacy of brief telephone psychotherapy with callers to a suicide hotline. Suicide Life Threat Behav. 2005 Jun;35(3):317-28.	3
263 Ricciardi A, McAllister V, Dazzan P. Is early intervention in psychosis effective? Epidemiologia e Psichiatria Sociale. 2008 Jul-Sep;17(3):227-35.	6
264 Richa N, Richa S, Salloum S, Baddoura C, Millet B, Mirabel-Sarron C. Familial risk factors influencing the course and the evolution of bipolar disorder: Literature review. Journal de Therapie Comportementale et Cognitive. 2009 Dec;19(4):141-5.	1
265 Rihmer Z, Akiskal H. Do antidepressants t(h)reat(en) depressives? Toward a clinically judicious formulation of the antidepressant-suicidality FDA advisory in light of declining national suicide statistics from many countries. Journal of Affective Disorders. 2006 Aug;94(1-3):3-13.	6
266 Rihmer Z, Gonda X. The Effect of Pharmacotherapy on Suicide Rates in Bipolar Patients. CNS Neurosci Ther. 2011 Aug 1.	6
267 Ritschel LA. Does mindfulness matter? investigating the effectiveness of an outpatient dialectical behavior therapy program. Dissertation Abstracts International: Section B: The Sciences and Engineering. 2006;67(6-B):3464.	3
268 Robertson HT, Allison DB. Drugs associated with more suicidal ideations are also associated with more suicide attempts. PLoS One. 2009;4(10):e7312.	9

Excluded Trials	Exclusion Code
269 Robinson DS, Gilmor ML, Yang Y, et al. Treatment effects of selegiline transdermal system on symptoms of major depressive disorder: a meta-analysis of short-term, placebo-controlled, efficacy trials. Psychopharmacol Bull. 2007;40(3):15-28.	6
270 Robinson J, Hetrick S, Gook S, et al. Study protocol: the development of a randomised controlled trial testing a postcard intervention designed to reduce suicide risk among young help-seekers. BMC Psychiatry. 2009;9(59).	6
271 Robinson J, Hetrick SE, Martin C. Preventing suicide in young people: systematic review. Aust N Z J Psychiatry. 2011 Jan;45(1):3-26.	7
272 Rodgers PL, Sudak HS, Silverman MM, Litts DA. Evidence-based practices project for suicide prevention. Suicide Life Threat Behav. 2007 Apr;37(2):154-64.	5
273 Rubino A, Roskell N, Tennis P, Mines D, Weich S, Andrews E. Risk of suicide during treatment with venlafaxine, citalopram, fluoxetine, and dothiepin: retrospective cohort study. BMJ. 2007 Feb 3;334(7587):242.	9
274 Rucci P, Frank E, Scocco P, et al. Treatment-emergent suicidal ideation during 4 months of acute management of unipolar major depression with SSRI pharmacotherapy or interpersonal psychotherapy in a randomized clinical trial. Depress Anxiety. 2011 Apr;28(4):303-9.	2
275 Russell G, Owens D. Psychosocial assessment following self-harm: Repetition of nonfatal self-harm after assessment by psychiatrists or mental health nurses. Crisis: The Journal of Crisis Intervention and Suicide Prevention. 2010;31(4):211-6.	9
276 Safer DJ, Zito JM. Do antidepressants reduce suicide rates? Public Health. 2007 Apr;121(4):274-7.	6
277 Sakinofsky I. Treating suicidality in depressive illness. Part 1: current controversies. Can J Psychiatry. 2007 Jun;52(6 Suppl 1):71S-84S.	7
278 Sakinofsky I. Treating suicidality in depressive illness. Part 2: does treatment cure or cause suicidality? Can J Psychiatry. 2007 Jun;52(6 Suppl 1):85S-101S.	7
279 Salvatore T. Peer specialists can prevent suicides. Behav Healthc. 2010 Oct;30(9):31-2.	6
280 Sambrook S, Abba N, Chadwick P. Evaluation of DBT emotional coping skills groups for people with parasuicidal behaviours. Behavioural and Cognitive Psychotherapy. 2007 Apr;35(2):241-4.	3
281 Sammet l, Brockmann J, Schauenburg H. Therapeutic intervention in suicidal states-- An empirical based case study on the basis of the Control-Mastery Theory. Forum der Psychoanalyse: Zeitschrift fur klinische Theorie & Praxis. 2007 Mar;23(1):18-32.	1
282 Schneeweiss S, Patrick AR, Solomon DH, et al. Comparative safety of antidepressant agents for children and adolescents regarding suicidal acts. Pediatrics. 2010 May;125(5):876-88.	9
283 Schneeweiss S, Patrick AR, Solomon DH, et al. Variation in the risk of suicide attempts and completed suicides by antidepressant agent in adults: a propensity score-adjusted analysis of 9 years' data. Arch Gen Psychiatry. 2010 May;67(5):497-506.	9
284 Scholz BA, Hammonds CL, Boomershine CS. Duloxetine for the management of fibromyalgia syndrome. J Pain Res. 2009;2:99-108.	6
285 Schumock GT, Lee TA, Joo MJ, Valuck RJ, Stayner LT, Gibbons RD. Association between Leukotriene-Modifying Agents and Suicide: What is the Evidence? Drug Saf. 2011 Jul 1;34(7):533-44.	7
286 Seemuller F, Lewitzka U, Muller HJ. In people taking antidepressants, suicidal behaviour is less common when they are taking them than in unexposed periods. Evid Based Ment Health. 2011 Nov;14(4):98.	6
287 Shern D. Examining costs and benefits in the health care debate. Psychiatric Services. 2009 Apr;60(4):419.	6
288 Simon GE, Savarino J, Operskalski B, Wang PS. Suicide risk during antidepressant treatment. Am J Psychiatry. 2006 Jan;163(1):41-7.	9

Excluded Trials	Exclusion Code
289 Simpson G, Franke B, Gillett L. Suicide prevention training outside the mental health service system: evaluation of a state-wide program in Australia for rehabilitation and disability staff in the field of traumatic brain injury. Crisis. 2007;28(1):35-43.	3
290 Singh T, Williams K. Atypical depression. Psychiatry. 2006 Apr;3(4):33-9.	3
291 Sinyor M, Levitt AJ. Effect of a barrier at Bloor Street Viaduct on suicide rates in Toronto: natural experiment. BMJ. 2010;341:c2884.	4
292 Siyez DM. Prevention of Suicides during Adolescence: A Review. Cocuk ve Genclik Ruh Sagligi Dergisi. 2005;12(2):92-101.	1
293 Skegg K, Herbison P. Effect of restricting access to a suicide jumping site. Aust N Z J Psychiatry. 2009 Jun;43(6):498-502.	4
294 Slee N, Garnefski N, van der Leeden R, Arensman E, Spinhoven P. Cognitive-behavioural intervention for self-harm: Randomised controlled trial. British Journal of Psychiatry. 2008 Mar;192(3):202-11.	2
295 Smith EG, Craig TJ, Ganoczy D, Walters HM, Valenstein M. Treatment of Veterans with depression who died by suicide: timing and quality of care at last Veterans Health Administration visit. J Clin Psychiatry. 2011 Sep 7;72(5):622-9.	5
296 Soomro GM. Deliberate self-harm (and attempted suicide). Clin Evid (Online). 2008;12:1012.	7
297 Spirito A, Simon V, Cancilliere MK, et al. Outpatient psychotherapy practice with adolescents following psychiatric hospitalization for suicide ideation or a suicide attempt. Clin Child Psychol Psychiatry. 2011 Jan;16(1):53-64.	3
298 Stanley B, Brown G, Brent DA, et al. Cognitive-behavioral therapy for suicide prevention (CBT-SP): treatment model, feasibility, and acceptability. Journal of the American Academy of Child and Adolescent Psychiatry. 2009 Oct;48(10):1005-13.	3
299 Stanley N, Mallon S, Bell J, Manthorpe J. Suicidal students' use of and attitudes to primary care support services. Primary Health Care Research and Development. 2010 Oct;11(4):315-25.	3
300 Stapleton J. Do the 10 UK suicides among those taking the smoking cessation drug varenicline suggest a causal link? Addiction. 2009 May;104(5):864-5.	6
301 Steele MM, Doey T. Suicidal behaviour in children and adolescents. Part 2: treatment and prevention. Can J Psychiatry. 2007 Jun;52(6 Suppl 1):35S-45S.	7
302 Stewart C, Rapp-Paglicci L, Rowe W. Evaluating the efficacy of the prodigy prevention program across urban and rural locales. Child & Adolescent Social Work Journal. 2009 Feb;26(1):65-75.	3
303 Stiffman AR, Brown E, Striley CW, Ostmann E, Chowa G. Cultural and Ethical Issues Concerning Research on American Indian Youth. Ethics & Behavior. 2005;15(1):1-14.	3
304 Stone M, Laughren T, Jones ML, et al. Risk of suicidality in clinical trials of antidepressants in adults: analysis of proprietary data submitted to US Food and Drug Administration. BMJ. 2009;339:b2880.	8
305 Takada M, Shima S. Characteristics and effects of suicide prevention programs: comparison between workplace and other settings. Ind Health. 2010;48(4):416-26.	7
306 Tarrier N, Taylor K, Gooding P. Cognitive-behavioral interventions to reduce suicide behavior: a systematic review and meta-analysis. Behav Modif. 2008 Jan;32(1):77-108.	3
307 Thomas SH, Drici MD, Hall GC, et al. Safety of sertindole versus risperidone in schizophrenia: principal results of the sertindole cohort prospective study (SCoP). Acta Psychiatrica Scandinavica. 2010 Nov;122(5):345-55.	2
308 Thuile J, Even C, Guelfi J. Mixed states in bipolar disorders: A review of current therapeutic strategies. L'Encephale: Revue de psychiatrie clinique biologique et therapeutique. 2005 Nov;31(5):617-23.	1

Excluded Trials	Exclusion Code
309 Tint A, Haddad PM, Anderson IM. The effect of rate of antidepressant tapering on the incidence of discontinuation symptoms: a randomised study. J Psychopharmacol. 2008 May;22(3):330-2.	3
310 Tondo L, Baldessarini RJ. Long-term lithium treatment in the prevention of suicidal behavior in bipolar disorder patients. Epidemiol Psichiatr Soc. 2009 Jul-Sep;18(3):179-83.	6
311 Tundo A, Cavalieri P, Navari S, Marchetti F. Treating bipolar depression - antidepressants and alternatives: A critical review of the literature. Acta Neuropsychiatrica. 2011 Jun;23(3):94-105.	7
312 Vaiva G, Ducrocq F, Meyer P, et al. Effect of telephone contact on further suicide attempts in patients discharged from an emergency department: randomised controlled study. BMJ. 2006 May 27;332(7552):1241-5.	2
313 Vaiva G, Walter M, Al Arab AS, et al. ALGOS: the development of a randomized controlled trial testing a case management algorithm designed to reduce suicide risk among suicide attempters. BMC Psychiatry. 2011;11:1.	6
314 van de Loo-Neus GH, Rommelse N, Buitelaar JK. To stop or not to stop? How long should medication treatment of attention-deficit hyperactivity disorder be extended? Eur Neuropsychopharmacol. 2011 Aug;21(8):584-99.	7
315 van den Bosch LM, Koeter MW, Stijnen T, Verheul R, van den Brink W. Sustained efficacy of dialectical behaviour therapy for borderline personality disorder. Behav Res Ther. 2005 Sep;43(9):1231-41.	2
316 van den Bosch LM, Verheul R. Patients with addiction and personality disorder: Treatment outcomes and clinical implications. Current Opinion in Psychiatry. 2007 Jan;20(1):67-71.	6
317 van der Feltz-Cornelis CM, Sarchiapone M, Postuvan V, et al. Best Practice Elements of Multilevel Suicide Prevention Strategies. Crisis. 2011 Sep 26:1-15.	7
318 van Wel EB, Bos EH, Appelo MT, Berendsen EM, Willgeroth FC, Verbraak MJ. [The efficacy of the systems training for emotional predictability and problem solving (STEPPS) in the treatment of borderline personality disorder. A randomized controlled trial]. Tijdschr Psychiatr. 2009;51(5):291-301.	1
319 von Knorring AL, Olsson GI, Thomsen PH, Lemming OM, Hulten A. A randomized, double-blind, placebo-controlled study of citalopram in adolescents with major depressive disorder. J Clin Psychopharmacol. 2006 Jun;26(3):311-5.	2
320 Wallin MT, Wilken JA, Turner AP, Williams RM, Kane R. Depression and multiple sclerosis: Review of a lethal combination. J Rehabil Res Dev. 2006 Jan-Feb;43(1):45-62.	6
321 Warner CH, Appenzeller GN, Parker JR, Warner C, Diebold CJ, Grieger T. Suicide prevention in a deployed military unit. Psychiatry. 2011 Summer;74(2):127-41.	5
322 Warner CH, Breitbach JE, Appenzeller GN, Yates V, Grieger T, Webster WG. Division mental health in the new brigade combat team structure: part II. Redeployment and postdeployment. Mil Med. 2007 Sep;172(9):912-7.	9
323 Weinberg I, Ronningstam E, Goldblatt MJ, Schechter M, Wheelis J, Maltsberger JT. Strategies in treatment of suicidality: identification of common and treatment-specific interventions in empirically supported treatment manuals. J Clin Psychiatry. 2010 Jun;71(6):699-706.	7
324 Weisler RH, Khan A, Trivedi MH, et al. Analysis of suicidality in pooled data from 2 double-blind, placebo-controlled aripiprazole adjunctive therapy trials in major depressive disorder. J Clin Psychiatry. 2011 Apr;72(4):548-55.	6
325 Wen B, Zhang Q-M, Li W-B. Effects of group counseling on depression and anxiety of patients with schizophrenia in rehabilitation. Chinese Mental Health Journal. 2006 Nov;20(11):762-4.	1

Excluded Trials	Exclusion Code
326 Wilcox HC, Kellam SG, Brown CH, et al. The impact of two universal randomized first- and second-grade classroom interventions on young adult suicide ideation and attempts. Drug Alcohol Depend. 2008 Jun 1;95 Suppl 1:S60-73.	4
327 Williams JM, Alatiq Y, Crane C, et al. Mindfulness-based Cognitive Therapy (MBCT) in bipolar disorder: preliminary evaluation of immediate effects on between-episode functioning. J Affect Disord. 2008 Apr;107(1-3):275-9.	3
328 Williams JM, Russell IT, Crane C, et al. Staying well after depression: trial design and protocol. BMC Psychiatry. 2010;10:23.	3
329 Wingate LR, Van Orden KA, Joiner TE, Jr., Williams FM, Rudd MD. Comparison of compensation and capitalization models when treating suicidality in young adults. J Consult Clin Psychol. 2005 Aug;73(4):756-62.	3
330 Wohlfarth TD, van Zwieten BJ, Lekkerkerker FJ, et al. Antidepressants use in children and adolescents and the risk of suicide. Eur Neuropsychopharmacol. 2006 Feb;16(2):79-83.	8
331 Woldu H, Porta G, Goldstein T, et al. Pharmacokinetically and clinician-determined adherence to an antidepressant regimen and clinical outcome in the TORDIA trial. Journal of the American Academy of Child & Adolescent Psychiatry. 2011 May;50(5):490-8.	3
332 Yerevanian BI, Koek RJ, Mintz J. Bipolar pharmacotherapy and suicidal behavior. Part I: Lithium, divalproex and carbamazepine. J Affect Disord. 2007 Nov;103(1-3):5-11.	9
333 Youssef NA, Rich CL. Does acute treatment with sedatives/hypnotics for anxiety in depressed patients affect suicide risk? A literature review. Annals of Clinical Psychiatry. 2008;20(3):157-69.	7
334 Zamorski MA. Suicide prevention in military organizations. Int Rev Psychiatry. 2011 Apr;23(2):173-80.	7
335 Ziemba KS, O'Carroll CB, Drazkowski JF, et al. Do antiepileptic drugs increase the risk of suicidality in adult patients with epilepsy?: a critically appraised topic. Neurologist. 2010 Sep;16(5):325-8.	7
336 Zisook S, Rush AJ, Lesser I, et al. Preadult onset vs. adult onset of major depressive disorder: a replication study. Acta Psychiatr Scand. 2007 Mar;115(3):196-205.	9